MW00513302

ESSENTIAL KETO BREAD COOKBOOK BUNDLE

Your Guide to Baking Low-Carb Bread. The Best Keto Bakers Cookbook With the Simple and Rapid Step by Step Recipes.

Dorothy Yosco

Sommario

KETO BREAD RECIPES

KETOGENIC RECIPES, QUICK AND EASY TO FOLLOW, TO BOOST YOUR ENERGY AND INTENSIFY YOUR WEIGHT LOSS.

Dorothy Yosco

What's A Keto Diet?

The keto diet plan is a really low-carb and higher-fat diet. It is like in many ways to additional low carb diets. Despite the fact that you eat much fewer carbs on a keto diet, then you keep moderate levels of protein ingestion and might raise your consumption of fatless. The decrease in carbohydrate intake places the body at a metabolic state called ketosis, in which fat, out of the diet plan and out of the entire body, is burnt for energy.

Exactly what "keto" signifies

Ketosis

Even the "keto" in a ketogenic diet includes from the simple fact that it permits the body to generate little gas molecules known as "ketones." This can be an alternate fuel source for your body, used if blood sugar (sugar) is in short supply. When you consume hardly any carbohydrates or not many calories, the liver also produces ketones from fat. These ketones subsequently function as a fuel supply through the human body, particularly for the brain. The mind is a hungry manhood which absorbs a great deal of energy daily, and it can not operate on fat straight. It may only run on sugar or ketones.

On a ketogenic diet, your body switches its fuel source to operate largely on burning, burning fat 24-7. If insulin levels become extremely low, fat burning may grow dramatically. It gets simpler to get into your fat stores to burn off them. This is excellent if you are attempting to get rid of weight, however, there may also be additional, less obvious advantages, for example less appetite and a continuous source of energy (minus the sugar levels and valleys we could gain from high carbohydrate foods). This can help you to stay focused and alert.

This is Something which is often reported by individuals to a keto diet [quite feeble signs].

The scientific support isn't powerful. Here are testimonials showing slight signs of developments:

European Journal of Clinical Nutrition 2013: Ketosis and appetite-mediating hormones and nutrients after weight reduction [randomized trial; moderate signs]

Neurobiology of Aging 2012: Dietary Ketosis improves memory in mild cognitive impairment [moderate signs for verbal memory enhancement in people with early Alzheimer's]

Epilepsy Research 2012: The consequences of the ketogenic diet in behavior and cognition. According to research, Cognitive Outcomes of a Ketogenic Diet on Neurocognitive Impairment in Illness Aging With HIV: A brand new study. [randomized trial; mild signs. After the body produces ketones, it passes a metabolic condition called ketosis. The quickest way to get there is by fasting -- maybe not ingesting anything but nobody could always fast eternally. Even a keto diet, on the flip side, also leads to ketosis and may be consumed forever. It's a lot of the advantages of fasting -- such as weight reduction -- without even needing to quickly long-term.

What to Eat on A Keto Diet

Listed below are normal foods to appreciate on a ketogenic diet. The amounts are net carbohydrates, i.e. digestible carbohydrates, per 100 g. To Stay in ketosis, lower is normally greater:

Keto diet food: Organic fats (olive, olive oil); Fish; Fish and fish; Eggs; Cheese; berries that grow above floor

What is the most important thing to do to achieve ketosis? Avoid eating a lot of carbohydrates. You may probably have to keep carbohydrate intake below 50 g daily of net carbohydrates, ideally under 20 g. The fewer carbohydrates, the more successful it seems to be for attaining ketosis, losing weight, or enhancing type two diabetes carbs can be useful in the beginning. But if you follow our preferred recipes and foods you are able to remain keto even without restricting.

Bakery Ketogenic Recipes

Miss bread and other baked products on low carbohydrate or keto? It is quite feasible to create, but it needs different ingredients and it is only... different. Here is our guide to low-fat ingredients, significant things to think about and all our best low-carb recipes!

How Does it Work

Keto baking makes utilization of cereal flour replacements that could offer Building, binding influence and a few of the performance given by wheat germ proteins (e.g. gas retention, visco-elasticity). Substitutes contain floor forms/flour of:

Exotic fruits and tree nuts such as almonds, pecans, walnuts, hazelnuts, cashews, macadamia nuts, and pistachios (freezing of powerful flavours may be required)
Coconut
Flax meal (whole gold flax seed)
Sunflower and pumpkin seeds
Garbanzo beans, chickpeas, sesame seeds, soy milk (freezing of tastes may be required)
Protein isolates and protein targets on pulses and legumes
Gums like xanthan gum and CMC
Collagen

Eggs
Casein, cocoa powder, cheese, milk solids

Formulation

The next keto bread formulation utilizes no yeast. Additionally, it includes no or low levels of sugars and damaged carbohydrates and amylases. In cases like this, steam creation during baking in addition to chemical-leaveners are accountable for bread loaf increasing and quantity develop.

Keto Bread Formula

Ingredients for Low-Carb Baking

Low-carb baking differs from traditional baking. To start with you want to get to understand a lot of fresh ingredients utilized instead of bread made from wheat or other grains. The most usual ones we use in this book are vanilla flour, coconut milk and earth psyllium husk powder.

Almond flour1 is really a gluten free nut flour which should include nothing but earth blanched almonds. This usually means you could create your own in the home, away from scratch, by milling whole blanched almonds into a nice meal (unless you only wish to purchase it). Employing a spice or coffee grinder normally works best. Take care not to grind them too long or the nuts may discharge their fat and also you 'll wind up with almond butter, that is a fantastic tasting nut butter although not exactly what you're going for when creating almond flour.

1 cup (240 ml) of wheat germ weighs 31/2 ounce. (99 g).

Coconut flour consists of Cold-pressed coconut flesh that has been dried and then ground into a nice meal. It's a feature coconut taste along with a high fiber material which contrasts the liquid within a dough. As it, such as almond milk, is fermented it will not create a soup increase like conventional pasta when yeast is included.

1 cup (240 ml) of coconut milk Weighs 41/2 ounce. (128 g).

Ground psyllium husk powder is 100 percent Pulverized psyllium husk cubes and can be utilized to provide a bread-like feel to what you are baking. As a result of the high fiber content it is frequently sold as a diuretic that could be useful to know in case you've got a sensitive digestive tract. When adding it into a liquid it becomes a gel-like material. It works somewhat like gluten in conventional baking, making it feasible to take care of the dough when forming or rolling it.

1 tbl of earth psyllium husk powder Weighs (10 g).

These products tend to disagree a Lot between various brands that makes low-fat baking somewhat catchy. By way of instance, some manufacturers of earth psyllium husk powder colour the bread purple. It does not appear to impact the flavor however, leaves the outcome somewhat longer... purple. The number of carbohydrates in coconut and almond flour may also change quite a difference between various brands. Read the labels and decide on the best one available.

Substituting flours

A frequent question is if you are able to Substitute almond milk for coconut milk as well as also the other way round. Yes, frequently you can although not in equal quantities. 1 cup of almond milk may be substituted for 1/3 cup of bread. 1/3 cup of coconut milk may be substituted for 2/3 cup almond milk + 1.5 tbsp of ground psyllium husk powder. The numbers might want to be corrected based upon what brands you are using.

Processing

Processing of keto bread can be very distinct from yeast-leavened bread created out of wheat-flour. The subsequent is a step by step keto baking process:

1. Ingredient scaling

2. Eggs prep and 1st blending. Separate the eggs and place the whites and cream of tartar in a large mixing bowl and blend on high speed till stiff peaks form.

3. 2nd Mixing. Mix egg yolk, almond Flour, butter, baking powder, salt, stevia, and 1/3 of those egg whites foam till a thick, uniform batter kinds.

4. Twist the foam. Fold in the rest Whipped egg whites in two parts.

5. Depositing or panning. Grease with Coconut oil spray before panning. An 8 x 4-inch loaf pan is generally utilized.

6. Baking. Given that the high density of this Formula, baking is performed in 400--420°F (204--216°C) into an internal temperature of 204°F (95°C). This typically requires 25--35 minutes. The more complicated the oven temperature, the longer the time.

7. Depanning

8. Cooling to loaf inner temperature of 95--105°F (35--40°C) prior packaging.

9. Packaging or functioning

Application

Keto baking is one form of fermented baking. This is because the majority of wheat germ substitutes and ingredients used in the creation of keto baked products come from fermented sources which don't belong to some Triticum species or alternative possibly gluten-containing cereals.

General guidelines:

- Mixing: it's essential to avoid any contamination of egg whites using butter since fat could create the egg to divide and reduce the capability to entrap atmosphere. Strict cleaning procedures such as gear, process tools and utensils must be carried out before beginning new batches.

- Baking: Vitamin profiling is a fantastic tool for controlling and monitoring the baking procedure. Given the radically different formulation in conventional bread, it's a good idea for optimum outcomes to comprehend the significance between oven ailments (timing/temperature) and microbial inactivation, crumb place and colour formation.

1.The Keto Bread

Smear with butter, and You'll think You're ingesting the real thing! Keto bread sport a pleasant crispy crust with a tender, wet centre. It is bread -- you understand exactly what to do. Savor it hot, straight from the toaster, or suspend, defrost, and toast to perfection...

Ingredients
- 5 tablespoons ground psyllium husk powder
- 1/4 cups almond milk
- 2 teaspoon baking powder
- 1 teaspoon sea salt
- 1 cup water
- 2 teaspoon cider vinegar
- 3 egg whites
- 2 tablespoons sesame seeds (optional)

Directions
- Preheat the oven at exactly 350°F.
- Add the dry ingredients in a big bowl. Bring the water to a boil.
- Add vinegar and egg whites into your dry ingredients, and blend well. Add boiling water, while hammering

using a hand mixer for approximately 30 minutes. Do not over mix the bread, the consequences should resemble Play-Doh.

- Wet hands with a little olive oil and then form dough into 6 distinct rolls. Put on a greased baking sheet. Top with discretionary sesame seeds.

- Bake on the lower rack in your oven for 50--60 minutes, based on how big your own bread rolls. They are done if you hear a hissing noise when tapping on the base of the bun.

- Serve with toppings and butter of your choice.

How much carbs does exactly the keto bread comprise?

The keto bread Includes 2 net carbs A bun (a comparable bun of frequent bread may comprise about 20 g of carbohydrates). That makes it a good choice to get a ketogenic diet. Expand the nourishment tab over for the entire nutrition facts.

Could I substitute ingredients?

In all baking, and particularly in low-carb, the ingredients and quantities used are significant. The eggs and earth psyllium husk are tough to substitute in this recipe. If you do not like almond milk or in case you have an allergy, then you are able to create this recipe with coconut oil flour instead. Substitute the quantity of almond milk to get a third as a lot of coconut milk and twice the amount of egg whites. For another appearance and some pinch, scatter seeds onto the buns until you pop them inside the oven -- poppy seeds, sesame seeds or not a few salt flakes and blossoms? Scrub your bread with your favorite seasoning to create them ideal for what you're serving these with. You are able to use garlic powder, crushed caraway seeds along with your own homemade bread seasoning.

2. Keto BLT with cloud bread

Can there be a more celestial flavor combo than bacon, tomato and lettuce? Only the mere mention of "BLT" along with the clouds begin to part! We paired with this mouthwatering, keto variant with fluffy cloud hosting, also referred to as oopsie bread. Oops, it is bread! Gluten-free along with grain-free, it is a heavenly low-carb spin on a timeless sandwich. Indulge.

Ingredients

- Cloud bread
- 3 eggs
- 4 oz. cream cheese
- 1 pinch salt
- 1/2 tbsp ground psyllium husk powder
- 1/2 teaspoon baking powder
- 1/4 teaspoon cream of tartar (optional)

Filling

4 tablespoons mayonnaise

5 oz. Bacon

2 oz. Lettuce

1 tomato, thinly chopped

Directions

Cloud bread

- Preheat oven to 300°F (150°C).
- Separate the eggs, with egg whites in 1 bowl and egg yolk into another. Notice that egg whites glow better at a metallic or ceramic bowl rather than plastic.
- Whip egg whites with salt (and cream of tartar, if you're utilizing any) until quite stiff, rather utilizing a hand-held mixer. You must be in a position to flip the bowl without the egg whites going.
- Add cream cheese, psyllium husk and baking powder and blend well.
- Fold the whites egg into the egg yolk mix -- attempt to keep the atmosphere in the egg whites.
- Put two dollops of this mixture per serving onto a paper-lined skillet. Spread the circles out using a spatula to approximately 1/2 inch (1 cm) thick bits.
- Bake for approximately 25 minutes, till they turn gold.

Building the BLT

- Fry the bacon in a skillet on moderate heat until crispy.
- Put the cloud bread bits top-side down.
- Spread mayonnaise on every bread.
- Put celery, lettuce and celery at layers involving the bread wedges.

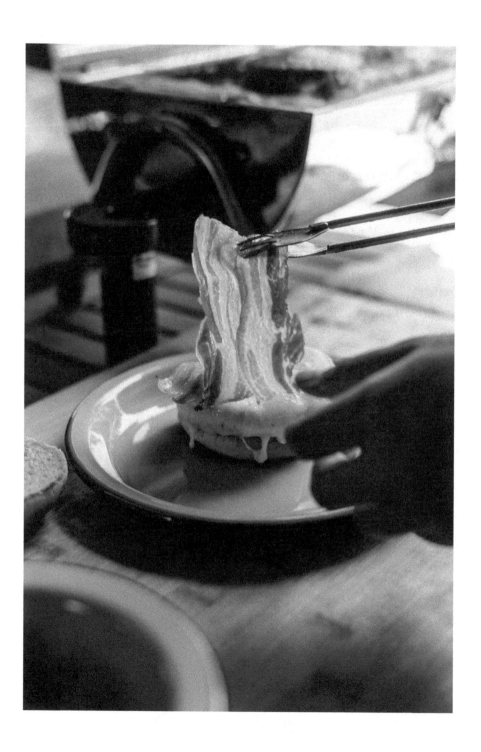

3. Keto naan bread with melted garlic

Do not skip the bread make your personal keto variant of naan for this particular one-of-a-kind recipe. After that, achieve supreme crave-worthiness together with all the garlic butter. Mmmmm...

Ingredients

Keto naan
- 3/4 cup coconut milk
- 2 tablespoons ground psyllium husk powder
- 1/2 tsp onion powder (optional)
- 1/2 teaspoon baking powder
- 1 teaspoon salt
- 1/3 cup roasted coconut oil
- 2 cups boiling water
- Coconut oil, for frying (optional)
- Sea salt

Garlic butter
- 4 oz. Butter
- 2 garlic cloves, minced

Directions

- Mix all dry ingredients to the keto naan at a bowl. Add lemon and oil water (hold any of it back if it is not required) and stir completely.

- Allow to rise to 5 minutes. The dough can turn business fairly fast, but remain flexible. It must resemble the consequences of Play-Doh. If you discover it is overly fussy then add psyllium husk till it seems right. When it's too firm, then add a number of the rest of the water. The sum required may change based on what kind of husk or coconut milk you use.

- Split into 6 or 8 pieces and shape into chunks which you sew together with your hands straight on parchment paper or even onto the kitchen countertops.

- Fry rounds at a skillet over moderate heat before the naan turn a nice gold colour. Based upon your skillet you are able to add a coconut oil into it so that the bread does not stick.

- Heat the oven to 140°F then keep the bread warm as you create more.

- Melt the butter and then stir into the freshly squeezed garlic. Use the melted butter on the bread bits utilizing a brush and then scatter flaked salt at top.

- Pour the remainder of the garlic butter into a bowl and dip pieces of bread in it.

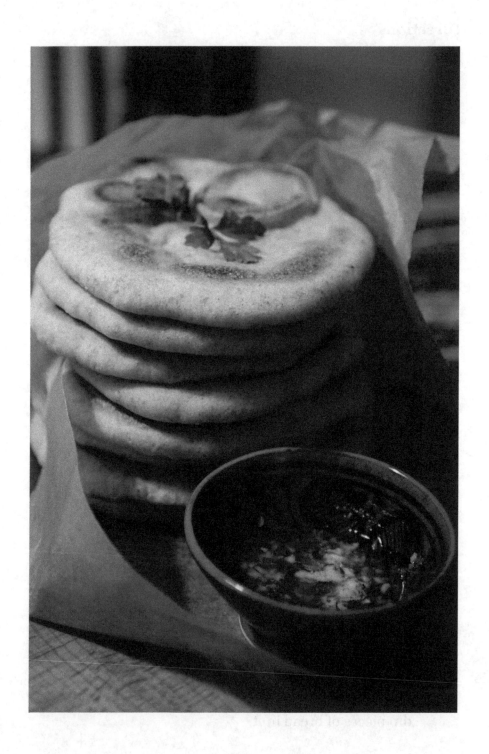

4. Keto garlic bread

This yummy keto bread could be served as an appetizer, a bite or as a side dish. It is crispy on the outside, soft on the inside and also has a beautiful taste as a result of its garlic butter. Only 1 gram of carbohydrates per slice.

Ingredients

Bread

- 11/4 cups almond milk
- 5 tablespoons ground psyllium husk powder
- 2 teaspoon baking powder
- 1 teaspoon sea salt
- 2 teaspoon cider vinegar or white wine vinegar
- 1 cup boiling water
- 3 egg whites

Garlic butter

- 4 oz. Butter at room temperature
- 1 garlic clove, minced
- 2 tablespoons fresh parsley, finely chopped
- 1/2 teaspoon salt
-

Directions

- Preheat the oven to 350°F exactly (175°C). Mix the ingredients to your bread into a bowl.

- Boil the water and then add the vinegar and egg whites into the bowl, even while stirring using a hand mixer for approximately 30 minutes. Do not overmix the dough the consequences should resemble Play-Doh.

- Form with wet hands to 10 pieces and roll up to hot dog buns. Be certain that you leave enough distance between them to the baking sheet to double in size.

- Bake on lower rack in oven for about 40-50 minutes, then they are done once you're able to hear a hissing noise when tapping on the base of the bun.

- Create the garlic butter whereas the bread is baking. Apply all of the ingredients together and place in the refrigerator.

- Simply take the buns from the oven when they are completed and leave to allow cool. Just take the garlic butter from the refrigerator. If the buns are chilled, cut them in halves, then with a serrated knife and distribute garlic butter on each half.

- Turn up your oven to 425°F (225°C) and inhale the garlic for 10-15 minutes, until golden brown.

If you do not enjoy almond milk or if You've got an allergy, so you are able to create this recipe with coconut oil flour instead. Substitute the Quantity of almond milk to get a third too a lot of coconut bread and Double the amount of egg whites.

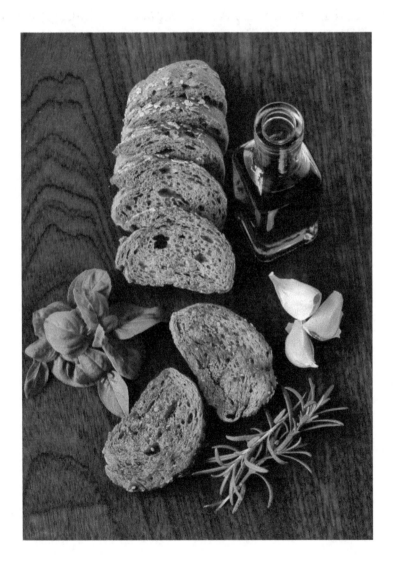

5. Keto mummy hot dogs

Succulent? Check. Savory? Check. A Little frightening? Check. Wrapping up these dogs in cheesy goodness makes dinner yummy and lively. Bonus: All these packs of chilling pleasure are keto too.

Ingredients

- 1/2 cup almond milk
- 4 tablespoons coconut flour
- 1/2 teaspoon salt
- 1 teaspoon baking powder
- Two 1/2 ounce. Butter
- 6 oz. shredded cheese
- 1 egg
- 1-pound sausages in hyperlinks, or uncured Hot dogs
- 1 egg, for cleansing the dough
- 16 tsp, for your mummies eyes (optional)

Directions
- Preheat your oven at exactly 350°F.
- Mix almond milk, coconut milk and baking powder in a big bowl.

- Melt the cheese and butter in a bowl on low heat. Stir thoroughly with a wooden spoon for a smooth and elastic batter. In few minutes, remove from heat.
- Pour the egg to the pasta mixture, then add the cheese mix, mixing all till it will become a firm dough.
- Flatten to a rectangle, roughly 8×14 inches (20×35 cm).
- Cut to 8 long strips, less than an inch wide (1.5--2 cm).
- Wrap the broth round the hot dog and then brush using a little egg.
- Insert your baking sheet lined with parchment paper and bake for 15--20 seconds before the dough is golden brown. The hot dog is going to be accomplished by then also.
- Push two tsp to every hot dog to make them seem like eyes but just for decoration. Do not eat the cloves!

Hint!

Using bigger hot dogs? Pre-fry them For a few minutes before wrap them up from the cheese and baking.

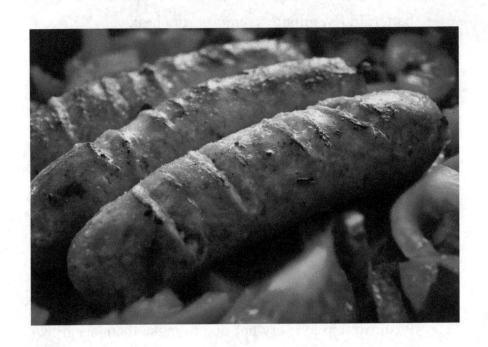

6. Soft keto seed bread

The following is a Fantastic keto bread choice, Baked with coconut and almond flour. It is compact and incredibly satisfying. A couple of pieces with lots of toppings can go quite a distance.

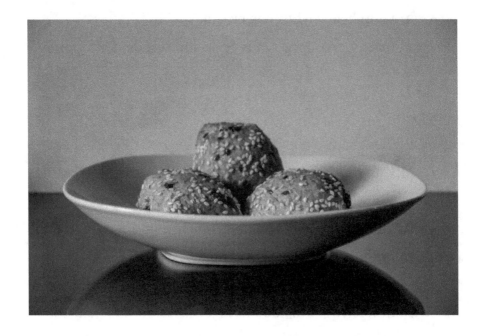

Ingredients

- 1 cup almond milk
- 3/4 cup coconut milk
- 1/3 cup sesame seeds
- 1/2 cup flaxseed

- 1/4 cup earth psyllium husk powder
- 3 teaspoon baking powder
- 1 teaspoon ground fennel seeds ground caraway seeds
- 1 teaspoon salt
- 7 oz. Cream cheese, at room temperature
- 6 eggs
- 1/2 cup of coconut oil or melted butter
- 3/4 cup heavy whipping cream
- 1 tablespoon poppy seeds or sesame seeds, for topping.

Directions

- Preheat your oven to 350°F that is (175°C).
- Mix all dry ingredients, except the seeds to the batting, in a bowl.
- In another bowl, toss all remaining ingredients till smooth.
- Insert the wet mixture into the dry mix and blend completely. Set the dough in a greased bread pan, about 4 x 5 inches (non stick or use parchment paper). Sprinkle the top with all the seeds.
- Bake for approximately 45 minutes about the lower rack from the oven. Prick the bread using a knife to find out if it's prepared, it must come out blank. Take it from the oven and take out the bread out of the shape.

- Remove the parchment paper and then allow the loaf cool on a rack. If the loaf is permitted to cool at the shape that the crust will be more pliable.
- Drink it baked along with your favourite toppings.

Serving suggestions

This bread is fantastic for toasting and May also be utilized to create your favorite sandwiches. Combine it with celery, tomato and lettuce to get an amazing BLT or function it as a side for your favorite low-carb or keto soup.

Storing the bread

This bread has to be stored from the refrigerator or in the freezer. Once kept in the refrigerator it retains up to five days. If you would like to keep it in the freezer we propose cutting on it prior to doing this. Put a little parchment paper between each piece to create single servings simpler. Thaw the bread from the refrigerator or in space temperature then toast it to optimal taste.

7. Keto bread twists

These decadent, wondrous twists are filled with yummy pesto taste. Mozzarella meets glowing herbs together with the pleasing, gold bread-like crust. Bite into those to get a fast keto bite or an ideal side dish. Or serve up to your dish of keto appetizers at the next cocktail party.

Ingredients

- 1/2 cup almond milk
- 1/4 cup coconut milk
- 1/2 teaspoon salt
- 1 teaspoon baking powder
- 1 egg, beaten
- 2 oz. Butter
- 61/2 ounce. Shredded cheese, rather mozzarella
- 1/4 cup green pesto
- 1 egg, beaten, for cleaning the very best

Directions

- Preheat the oven at exactly 350°F.
- Apply all dry ingredients in a bowl. Add the egg and then mix.

- Melt the butter and the cheese together into a pot on low heat. Stir until the batter is smooth.
- Gradually insert the butter-cheese batter into the dry mix bowl and combine together into a firm dough.
- Set the dough on parchment paper is the extent of a square cookie sheet. Use a rolling pin and earn a rectangle, roughly 1/5-inch (5 mm) thick.
- Spread pesto on the top and cut to 1-inch (2.5 cm) strips. Twist them and put on a baking sheet lined with parchment paper. Brush spins with the whisked egg.
- Bake in the oven for 15--20 minutes till they're golden brown.

Suggestion!

If a dough appears to be sticky, place between 2 sheets of parchment paper prior to using the rolling pin. As soon as you've wrapped it out, remove the top bit of parchment paper. If you're experiencing difficulty twisting, or need a different look in the twist, then use a cookie cutter to cut out two identical contours and then spread the pesto between, like a cookie or sandwich filling. Put to the parchment and inhale.

From pesto? No issue. Sub in almost any of your favorite spices. Paprika powder, curry, coriander, cumin or herbs such as thyme, peppermint and peppermint work nicely. Or have a grilled cheese filling with substituting a little bit of shredded cheese rather than pesto. For a modest additional selection, consider substituting a tiny parmesan for a number of these mozzarella.

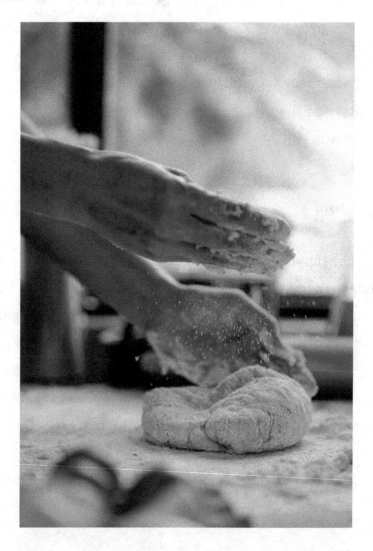

8. Keto pizza crust

Ingredients

- 11/4 cups almond milk
- 1/4 cup unflavored protein powder
- 4 tablespoons ground psyllium husk powder
- 1/2 teaspoon salt
- 2 tablespoon grated parmesan cheese
- 1 tablespoon Italian seasoning
- 2 teaspoon baking powder
- 2 eggs
- 1 cup of boiling water
- 3 tablespoons coconut oil or melted butter, for cleaning.

Directions

- Preheat the oven at exactly 375°F.
- In a skillet, combine the dry ingredients until well mixed. Add the eggs, stirring till well blended.
- Gradually add boiling water into the mix, before the dough thickens. Shape the dough into a ball using your hands.
- Set the ball onto a greased baking sheet. Spray a bit of parchment with oil and set it on top of the dough that

will simply disperse it. Utilize your hands or a rolling pin to spread the dough to a 16-inch round.

- The dough will grow to 2-3 times its own size, so produce the thickness one third of everything you desire the last crust to become.

- Put in oven and bake for exactly 25 minutes.

- Remove crust from oven and brush with coconut oil or butter and then return to oven. Broil for 3-8 minutes until the crust is crispy. Watch carefully in this measure to be certain that it doesn't burn off, but only crisps up. Start broiling using the crust flipped to clear the ground first. After that, turn it and then broil the very best.

- Let cool and store in the freezer till you would like to utilize it. If you cannot wait patiently add toppings and simmer for another 5-10 minutes until the cheese is melted and begins to brown.

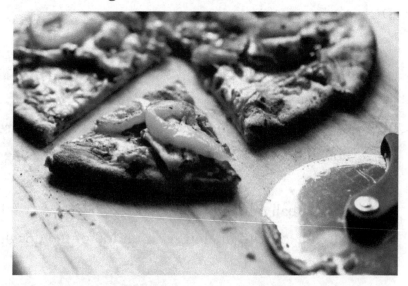

9. Keto coconut-flour bread

We called this one "Nearly Cornbread." However... well... no corn. Do not let this prevent you by pairing it with chili. Or spread the butter thick and pour it up with a large bowl of bone broth. Primal satisfaction!

Ingredients

- 1/2 cup coconut milk
- 1/4 teaspoon sea salt
- 1/4 teaspoon baking powder
- 6 eggs
- 1/2 cup roasted coconut oil

Directions

- Preheat the oven at exactly 350°F.
- Put in a medium sized bowl, sift together the dry skin.
- Simply apply the wet ingredients to the dry ingredients and then stir fry till quite smooth.
- Grease a little bread pan and then fill in 2/3 of how full of batter. Bake for about 50 minutes.

Tips

This bread is also neutral in taste but If you'd like to you can include your favorite spices or not attempt 1-2 tbsp of our vacation bread seasoning?

Storing

You can keep this bread at the Refrigerator for 3-4 days in the freezer up to 3 weeks. Ensure that you slice the bread before freezing it and then put parchment paper between each piece. This way you can always have easy 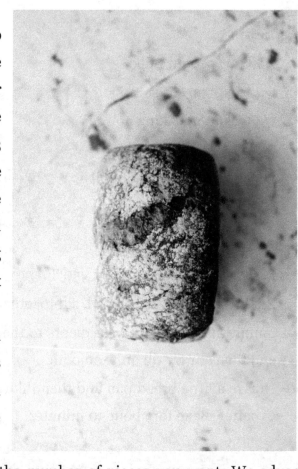 accessibility to the number of pieces you want. We advocate having a toaster or toaster oven.

10. Keto dosa

Dosa is a fermented Indian crepe created with lentils and rice. It is served with a gentle coconut chutney, plus it is among the very popular breakfast foods in the nation. This keto variant replaces the initial ingredients with almond milk, almond milk and cheese.

Ingredients

Keto dosa

- 1/2 cup almond milk
- 11/2 ounce. mozzarella cheese, shredded
- 1/2 cup almond milk
- 1/2 tsp ground cumin
- 1/2 tsp ground coriander seed
- salt, to taste

Directions

- In a bowl blend together all of the ingredients.
- Heat and lightly oil a skillet. It is extremely important to utilize a skillet to protect against the dosa from adhering to the pan.

- Pour the batter and then spread it round by shifting the pan. You wish to create a round form.
- Cook the dosa onto a very low heat. The cheese will begin to melt down and crisp up.
- When it is cooked all of the way through and also the dosa has become fine and golden brown on the other side fold it with the spatula.
- Evacuate from the pan and serve with coconut chutney.

Preparation:

Stir the coconut flesh, ginger, salt and fresh chilli in a food processor or even a mortar and pestle. Insert as much water as necessary to guarantee the mix is not too dry and much more moist such as a chutney.

Heat the coconut oil in a bowl combined Using the dried red chilli, mustard seeds, cumin seeds and curry leaves.

When the oil is warm as well as the mustard Seeds are popping include the floor chutney mix to the pan and turn off the cooker.

Mix everything well and then move into a bowl.

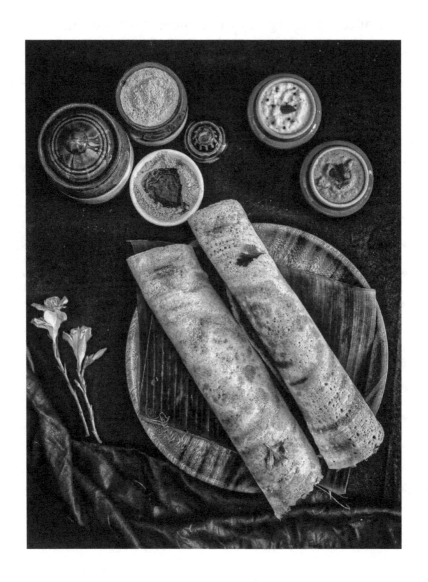

11. Nut-free keto bread

When you've nut allergies or only need a switch, this yummy low-carb bread is nut-free and tastes good, particularly toasted. Try it with mashed avocado, carrot eggs, melted cheese or other preferred toppings. Ideal for breakfast or any other meal.

Ingredients

- 6 eggs
- 12 ounces. shredded cheese
- 1 ounce. cream cheese
- 2 tablespoons ground psyllium husk powder
- 3 teaspoon baking powder
- 1/2 cup oat fiber
- 1/2 teaspoon salt
- 1 tablespoon butter, melted

Topping
- 3 tablespoon sesame seeds
- 2 tablespoon poppy seeds

Directions
- Preheat the oven at exactly 360°F.

- Whisk the eggs into a bowl. Add the cheese and the remaining ingredients, but for the butter and blend thoroughly.
- Grease a bread pan (8.5" x 4.5" x 2.75", garnished or garnished with parchment paper) using butter. Spread the dough out from the bread pan using a spatula.
- Spread the bread with sesame seeds and poppy seeds. Bake the bread for 35 seconds.
- Allow the bread cool. Slice and Revel in.

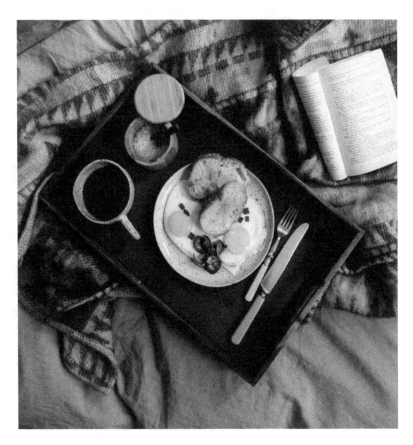

12. Keto English muffins

A flat bread made out of just three Ingredients including eggs, coconut milk and baking powder. Fantastic for breakfast or even the kids' lunch boxes.

Ingredients

- 2 eggs
- 2 tablespoon coconut flour
- 1/2 teaspoon baking powder
- 1 pinch salt
- 3 tablespoons butter or coconut oil, also for frying

Directions

- Mix with coconut milk, baking soda and a pinch of salt in a bowl.
- Crack the eggs to the bowl and whisk together. Let sit a couple of minutes.
- Put three dollops of this batter in a skillet with melted butter, on medium high.
- Turn the noodles following a few minutes and then fry a few more.
- Serve with butter and your favorite topping.
-

Suggestion!

You may as well bake them in the oven for approximately ten minutes in 400°F (200°C) at a well-greased cupcake tin (approximately 3 inches in diameter). They'll be like bread, but reduced in fat.

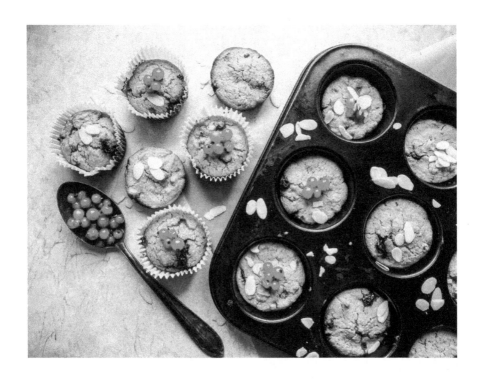

13. Keto French toast

Who does not enjoy a comfy brunch with a few French toast? We have adapted this hot classic to match all keto requirements. We are not skimping on the butter or cinnamon either. Enjoy!

Ingredients
- Mug bread
- 1 teaspoon butter
- 2 tablespoon almond milk
- 2 tablespoon coconut flour
- 11/2 teaspoon baking powder
- 1 pinch salt
- 2 eggs
- 2 tablespoon heavy whipping cream

Batter
- 2 eggs
- 2 tablespoon heavy whipping cream
- 1/2 tsp ground cinnamon
- 1 pinch salt
- 2 tablespoon butter

Directions

- Grease a huge mug or a glass dish with a flat base with butter.
- Mix with dry ingredients at the mug using a spoon or fork. Publish in the egg and then stir into the cream. Blend until smooth and make certain that there aren't any lumps.
- Microwave on high (roughly 700 g) for two minutes. Assess whether the bread has been completed at the center -- if microwave for another 15-30 minutes.
- Let cool and remove out of your mug. Slice in half an hour.
- Put in a bowl or freezer, whip together the egg, cream and cinnamon with a pinch of salt. Pour over the bread pieces and allow them to get soaked. Switch them around several times so that the bread pieces consume up to the egg mix as you can.
- Fry in a lot of butter and serve immediately.

Suggestion!

This recipe is based on our own Low-carb Tasting bread, however you may use some other low carb bread you would like.

If you do not need to Assess the dry Ingredients each moment, prepare your very own baking mixture beforehand. Take 10 tbsp (150 ml) almond milk, 10 tbsp (150 ml) coconut milk, 1 tsp salt and 2 ½ tsp baking powder. Then you've got the dry mixture prepared for 10 bits.

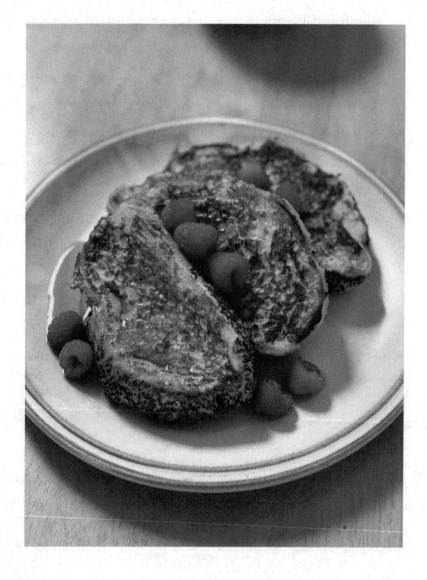

14. Soft keto tortillas

Soft, elastic, chewy keto tortillas Without nuts or legumes? Yes please! This dough works out like a conventional tortilla recipe and it cooks up into toasty rounds that are fantastic for filling with your favorite taco disperse goodies.

Ingredients

- 1 cup coconut milk
- 1/4 teaspoon baking soda
- 1/2 teaspoon salt
- 1/4 cup earth psyllium husk powder
- 1/2 cup of coconut oil
- 3 large egg whites
- 11/2 cups warm water

Directions

- Heat a big cast iron skillet or griddle moderate heat.
- In a big bowl, sift together the coconut bread, baking soda and salt. Whisk from the psyllium husk.
- Drizzle in the oil gradually as you stir the mixture, it is going to get moist and crumbly. Fold in the egg whites.

- Mix from the hot water cup at a time, ensuring it is completely mixed before adding water. Blend until the dough feels and looks just like moist play-doh.
- Twist 12 even-sized balls. Flatten the balls involving parchment paper onto a tortilla press or utilize a 6" pot and push down them.
- Cook two tortillas at one time on the massive griddle by lying horizontal to the hot, thick cast iron plus toasting 3 minutes per side, turning once. Put aside until all the tortillas are finished.

Suggestion!

If your mixture is moist add in 1 Teaspoon of psyllium husk at one moment, waiting a moment before blending in the subsequent one to make certain it's consuming liquid. Instead, if your mixture is too wet, add 1 tsp of water at a period in precisely the exact same manner until the perfect texture is accomplished, damp play-doh. Store the leftover tortillas by wrap up air and flat freezing and tight. To thaw toast hot cast iron.

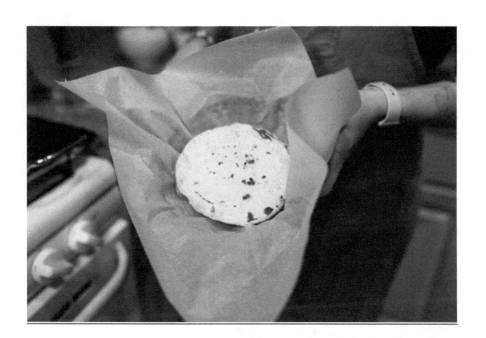

15. Keto bagels

Crispy on the outside, tender around the inside. Easy and flavorful seedy bagels, only waiting for you to include your favorite fillings.

Ingredients

Bagels

- 7 oz. mozzarella cheese
- 1 ounce. cream cheese
- 11/2 cups almond milk
- 2 teaspoon baking powder
- 1 egg

Topping

- 2 tsp flaxseed
- 1 teaspoon sesame seeds
- 1/2 teaspoon sea salt
- 1/4 tsp poppy seeds
- 1 egg

Directions

- Preheat the oven to 430°F (220°C) plus a large baking dish with parchment paper.

- Put the mozzarella and cream cheese in a medium microwave safe bowl and microwave on high for 1 second. Remove and stir fry. Duplicate in 30 second bursts until the cheese has melted and can be readily combined.
- In another bowl, whisk together the almond milk and baking powder, then until well blended. Insert the vanilla and egg milk mixture, into the melted cheese. Mix well until a smooth dough form. Kneading it onto a non stick surface, assists with this procedure!
- Split the dough into as many ingredients as pieces from the recipe, and then shape into bun contours. Put in your own lined baking tray.
- Take advantage of your hands, or even the use of a wooden spoon, then to shove a hole at the middle of every bun then shape it further till you've bagel contours.
- Set the seeds and simmer to your right mix right into a little bowl and then give it a quick stir to blend.
- Crack the next egg into a bowl and beat till blended.
- Brush top of each bagel liberally using the cherry then sprinkle with your correct mix.
- Bake in the oven for approximately 15 minutes

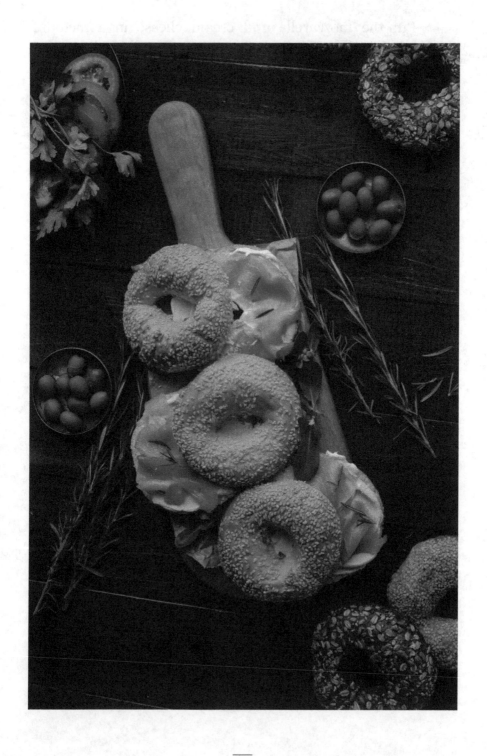

16. Low-carb tasting bread

Newly baked bread at 5 minutes? You have gotta be mesmerized... following is a slice of great news: it is accurate and it is low-carb and crispy, only how it's supposed to be. This recipe was circulating the web for some time today and turned into a quick low-carb classic. Learn exactly what all the fuss is all about!

Ingredients

- 1 tablespoon butter
- 1 tablespoon almond milk
- 1 tablespoon coconut flour
- 3/4 teaspoon baking powder
- 1/2 tsp poppy seeds
- 1 pinch salt
- 1 egg, beaten
- 1 tablespoon heavy whipping cream

Directions

- Add the butter from the mug (using a level underside) plus microwave.

- Mix together all dry ingredients into a bowl. Crack in the egg, then add the peanut butter and stir into the cream. Blend until smooth and make certain that there aren't any lumps.
- Pour the batter into the spool and then microwave on high (roughly 700 g) for two minutes. Assess whether the bread has been completed at the center -- if microwave for another 15-30 minutes.
- Let cool and remove out of your mug. Slice in half and toast -- that is the way you find the ideal texture and flavor.

Directions for baking in the oven
- Preheat oven to 350°F (175°C), also dirt a 4.5" wide, oven proof bowl.
- Put in a medium sized bowl, whisk together all dry ingredients, including the discretionary poppy seeds. Add the cream and egg, whisking until smooth. Make certain that there aren't any lumps. Pour the batter to the bowl.
- Put bowl in the oven and simmer for 10-15 minutes. Add a toothpick or sharp knife at the center of bread. If the toothpick is clean, it's done!
- Let cool and remove the bread out of the bowl. Slice in half and toast - that is the way you find the ideal texture and flavor

Prepare beforehand

For best results, prepare every piece individually. In the event you do not need to assess the dry ingredients each time you bake, then don't hesitate to prepare your very own baking mix beforehand. Take 10 tbsp (150 ml) almond milk, 10 tbsp (150 ml) coconut milk, 1 tsp salt and two 1⁄2 tsp baking powder. Then you've got the dry mixture prepared for 10 bits. Utilize 2 generous tbsp for every bit of bread.

Storing the bread

Feel free to create a few bits once you get cooking. You're able to continue to keep the unbaked dough from the fridge for 2-3 times or you may even freeze the mix. It will thaw in a couple of minutes in room temperature.

Flavoring

For extra flavor, year the bread with garlic or onion powder, also spices or herbs such as floor fennel and lavender. Additionally, it is wonderful with poppy, chia, hemp, or sesame seeds. Utilize about 1⁄2 tsp of seasoning to every slice.

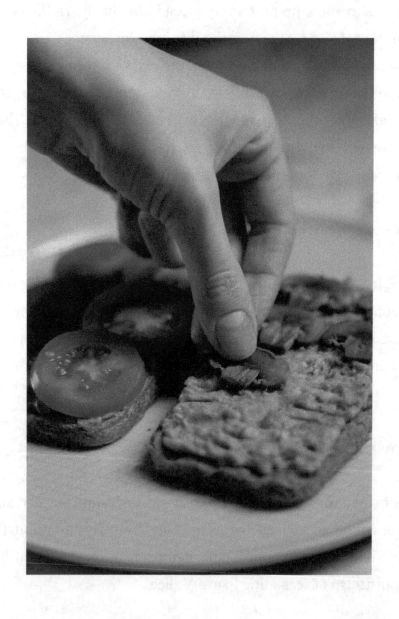

17. Keto cornbread

The love of cornbread is marginally regional, but it is universally adored. Possessing a tasty keto alternative is quite a treat. This variant has a crisp crust, and also a gentle, but rough crumb.

Ingredients

- 1/4 cup coconut milk
- 1⁄3 cup oat fiber
- 1⁄3 cup whey protein isolate
- 11/2 teaspoon baking powder
- 1/4 teaspoon salt
- 4 oz. Butter, melted
- 1⁄3 cup of bacon fat or coconut oil, melted
- 1/4 cup water
- 4 eggs
- 1/4 teaspoon corn extract (optional)

Directions

- Preheat oven to 350°F (175°C). Put a greased 10-inch (25 cm) cast iron skillet from the oven to warm as you make the cornbread.
- Blend all ingredients in a bowl.

- Add the melted butter, celery, celery, eggs, and water. Beat with a hand mixer. Stir in the corn infusion.
- Pour the cornbread mix into the hot cast iron skillet and bake for approximately 18 - 20 minutes till lightly browned and firm to the touch.

Suggestion!

The corn infusion is discretionary, but provides a more genuine, corn-like taste. If you do not have a cast iron skillet, then a pie tin or little oven-proof skillet will get the job done.

Whey protein isolate contains casein and Insulin eliminated and really isn't the like whey protein, that can be quite insulinogenic. Please check the ingredients whey protein isolate to be certain that there are not any additional sweeteners. Oat fiber is your pure insoluble fiber from the outer husk of the oat. As it isn't digestible, it doesn't affect blood sugar.

Storing

You can keep this bread in the refrigerator for up to five times. I you need to suspend it, it is possible to do this for as many as 3 weeks. We recommend cutting on it and putting parchment paper between for simple accessibility to the ideal quantity.

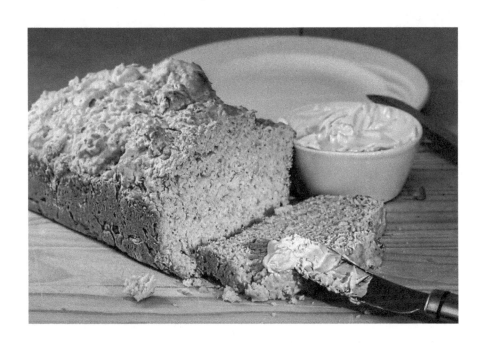

18. Keto golden sesame bread

Golden. Soft. Airy. Everything you Desire at a keto loaf. Additionally, the crowning touch sesame seeds. Try out this bread with hot stews, gratins or not... a fast sandwich. It is fermented and super simple to create!

Ingredients

- 4 eggs
- 7 oz. cream cheese
- 2 tablespoon sesame oil
- 2 tbsp mild olive oil, also more for brushing
- 1 cup almond milk
- 2 tablespoons ground psyllium husk powder
- 1 teaspoon salt
- 1 teaspoon baking powder
- 1 tablespoon sesame seeds
- Sea salt (optional)

Directions

- Preheat oven to 400°F (200°C).
- Beat cream cheese till fluffy. Add eggs, coconut oil and olive oil, then mix until well blended.
- Add remaining ingredients except for the seeds.

- Spread the dough into a baking tray (9" x 5" or 23 x 13 cm) garnished with butter lined with parchment paper. Let stand for 5 minutes.
- Brush with olive oil and then sprinkle with sesame seeds and a bit of sea salt.
- Bake for 25-30 minutes till golden brown at the top and never doughy in the center.

Suggestion!

You can save the bread from the refrigerator for 2-3 days slice it and then freeze for later usage. Reheat on reduced temperatures in the microwave or oven. You may also use the toaster to get extra crispness. If you're interested in finding a superb dish to choose the bread, then try our Turkish roasted beans recipe. Yum!

Perhaps not a lover of seeds? don't hesitate to sub in poppy seeds or flaxseeds.

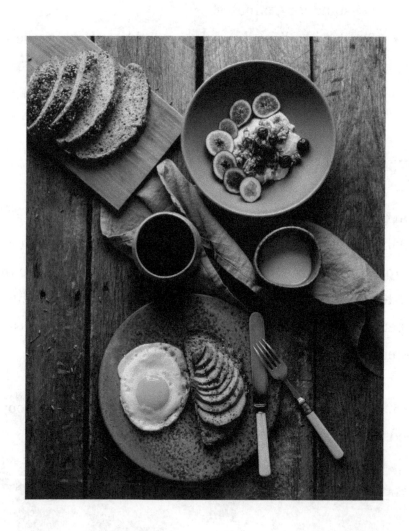

19. Paleo bread

Heads up, nut and seed fans -- this loaf's for you! Crunchy. Hearty. Oh-so-tasty. Additionally, it is keto, dairy-free and fermented. A complete pick for sandwiches, but delicious as a negative dish standalone snack. Do not forget the butter.

Ingredients
- 7 oz. almonds or hazelnuts
- 7 oz. Pumpkin seeds
- 3 oz. flaxseed
- 3 oz. sesame seeds
- 4 oz. sunflower seeds
- 2 oz. pecans or walnuts
- 1 tablespoon fennel seeds, crushed
- 2 tsp salt
- 6 eggs
- 1/3 cup melted coconut oil
- 1/2 teaspoon white wine vinegar (optional)

Directions
- Preheat the oven at exactly 300°F (150°C). Add your dry ingredients in a big bowl.
- Crack in your eggs. Add vinegar and oil. Mix well.
- Set the dough at a non stick or bread pan, approximately 5 x 10 inches (12 x 24 cm). Bake for one hour. Switch off

the heat and permit the bread to fully cool with the oven door ajar.

Suggestion!

This recipe creates an oversize loaf. Then keep in the fridge for up to weekly. Additionally, it adheres well; for optimal results, cut into thin pieces before freezing.

Spread a generous quantity of butter every piece --it'll be nearly as satiating as a complete meal!

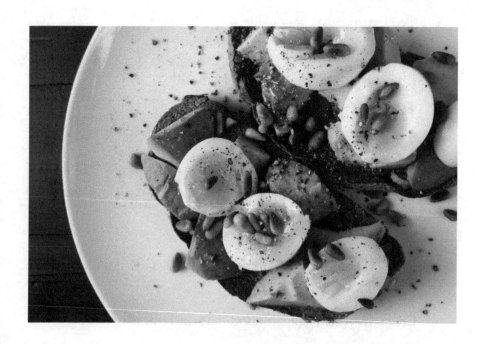

20. Low-carb cloud bread

Cloud bread (also Called oopsie Bread) is another superb low-carb bread choice. It is a flexible "bread" with no carbohydrates and may be consumed in many different means. You can get this as a sandwich as a bun to get a hotdog or hamburger.

Ingredients

- 3 eggs
- 41/2 ounce. cream cheese
- 1 pinch salt
- 1/2 tbsp ground psyllium husk powder
- 1/2 teaspoon baking powder
- 1/4 teaspoon cream of tartar (optional)

Directions

- Separate the eggs with the egg whites in 1 bowl and the egg yolks into another.
- Whip egg whites with salt until very stiff. You must be in a position to flip the bowl without the egg whites going.
- Mix the egg yolk and also the cream cheese nicely. If you'd like, include the psyllium seed husk and coconut powder (making it increasingly bread-like).

- Carefully fold the white egg into the egg yolk mixture -- attempt to keep the atmosphere in the egg whites.
- Put as many dollops of the mix as portions from the recipe onto a paper-lined baking tray. Spread the circles out using a spatula to approximately 1/2 inch (1 cm) thick bits.
- Bake in your oven at exactly 300° F for approximately 25 minutes -- till they turn gold.

The Way to store cloud bread

You are able to save the bread in the fridge for 2-3 days or in freezer for up to 3 weeks. Set a layer of parchment paper between every bread to steer clear of the bits sticking together. This way you are able to catch as many bits as you need and there is no need to thaw all of them at one time.

You are able to thaw frozen bread at room temperature or in the fridge. They taste much better if you toast them but you might also reheat them from the oven. Preheat the oven at exactly 300°F and then put the cloud bread bits onto the rack for approximately 5 minutes. They'll be new and good as brand new!

The best way to utilize potato bread

You can use this bread because the foundation for your favourite sandwich or utilize it like a hotdog or hamburger bun. There are actually no limitations so don't hesitate to change the toppings following your own personal preference.

The best way to change the bread recipe

This recipe does not have a great deal of Taste by itself making it good to use as sandwich bread. You are able to add a pinch by utilizing different types of seeds. You're able to use poppy seeds, sesame or sunflower seeds or another kind you prefer. Spread it on the bread until you inhale them. You are able to substitute roasted cream cheese, mascarpone cheese or calcium-rich Greek yogurt to your cream cheese. The very first option will provide you more taste and others more fluff, based on what you are opting for.

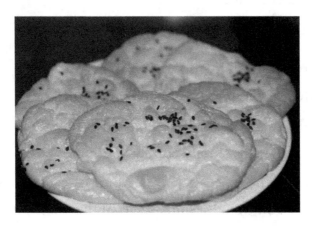

21. Fast low-carb bread

Sesame and citrus seeds make for some Nutty flavored low-fat flat bread that's the best foundation for your favorite spread or an open-faced sandwich. This recipe is easy and quick, with just two grams of carbohydrates per serving, also ends in a crispy yet tender fermented low-carb bread. Low-carb recipe.

Ingredients

- 2 oz. cream cheese
- 2 egg whites
- 2 tsp ground psyllium husk powder
- 1/2 cup almond milk
- 1/2 cup sesame seeds
- 1/4 cup sunflower seeds
- 11/2 teaspoon baking powder
- 2 pinches salt

Directions

- Preheat oven to 400°F (200°C).
- Mix egg whites and cream cheese in a bowl.
- Add remaining ingredients and function into the egg batter. Let rest for a couple of minutes.
- Shape the batter squares, you per serving. Sprinkle a little additional sesame seeds at the top if you prefer.

- Bake in oven 10--12 minutes till golden brown.
- Let them cool a little before appreciating them along with your favorite topping.

Tips!

If you do not need to get doughy Palms, spread the batter by means of a spatula to a greased baking dish, roughly 1 x 11 inch (20 × 30 cm). Cut the bread into bits later baking.

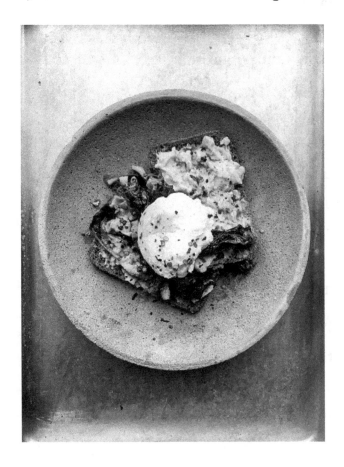

22. Low-carb poppy-seed bread

A filling sandwich having a tasty Low-carb bread with cottage cheese and poppy seeds, simple to create. Best with leafy greens along with a chicken curry salad!

Ingredients

Low-carb bread

- 8 oz. Cottage cheese
- 3 eggs
- 1 tablespoon olive oil
- 4 tablespoons chia seeds flaxseed
- 4 tablespoon sunflower seeds
- 1 teaspoon baking powder
- 1 teaspoon ground psyllium husk powder
- 1 teaspoon sea salt
- 1 tablespoon poppy seeds

Directions
- Mix all of the dry ingredients. Stir in eggs, cottage cheese and oil. Let sit 15 minutes.

- Distribute the batter onto a baking sheet lined with parchment paper. Bake in the oven at 350°F (175°C) to get 20--25 minutes.
- Let dry on a stand with no parchment paper.
- Cut to 6--8 serving pieces and love with butter and lettuce.
- Place the leftover bread from the refrigerator or freezer, so it is going to be just like freshly baked at the toaster.
- We've selected to serve the bread with a salad, a filling curry mayonnaise.

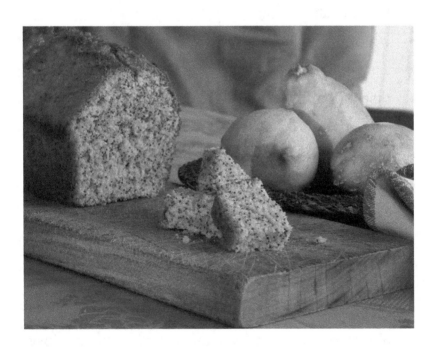

23. Keto "Bacon and Cheese" Zucchini Bread Recipe

This simple, moist Bacon and Cheese Keto Zucchini Bread recipe is ideal for brunch. It is best served warm topped with butter.

Ingredients

- 3 oz (1 cup) of Almond Flour
- 2 oz (1/2 cup) of Coconut Flour
- 1 tsp of Salt
- 1/2 tsp of Pepper
- 2 tsp of Baking Powder
- 1 tsp of Xanthan Gum
- 5 Eggs
- 2/3 cup of yoghurt, melted
- 4 oz (1 cup) Of Cheddar Cheese, grated
- 6 oz (1 cup) of Zucchini, grated and liquid thrown out
- 6 oz (1 cup) of Bacon, diced

Directions

- Preheat oven into 175C/350F.
- In a large bowl add the almond milk, coconut vinegar, pepper, salt, baking powder and xanthan gum. Mix well.
- Add the eggs and melted butter and blend well.

- Twist through 3/4 of this cheddar, alongside the zucchini and celery.
- Spoon to a greased 9in ceramic noodle dish (when using a metallic dish line with parchment paper) and simmer for 35 minutes, then remove from the oven and top with the cheese.
- Bake for another 10-15 minutes, until the cheese has browned and a skewer comes out clean.

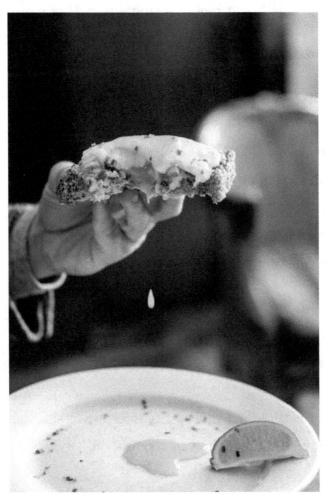

- Leave to cool for 20 minutes.
- Slice into 12 pieces and revel in warm.

24. Carb Bread

Ideal for keto egg whites, Low-carb grilled cheeses, as well as miniature French toasts, you will only require a couple of pantry staples to the ingredients, very similar to a number of the recipes within this listing. And that usually means you most likely already have everything you want on hand to check it out now. Although this bread makes a single part, it is possible to turn it in a loaf to feed your whole family due to this recipe.

Ingredients

- 2 tbsp almond milk
- 1/2 tbsp coconut flour
- 1/4 tsp baking powder
- 1 egg
- 1/2 tbsp peanut butter or ghee
- 1 tbsp unsweetened milk choice

Directions

- Add all the ingredients in a little bowl and whisk until smooth.
- Grease a three ×3-inch glass microwave-safe bowl or mould with butter, ghee, or coconut oil.

- Pour your mixture in to your well-greased bowl mold and microwave on high for 90 minutes.
- Gently remove your bread out of your glass dish or mould.
- Slice, toast, and melt butter at the top, if wanted

Tips

If you do not have a microwave, then attempt Skillet the dough at a small butter, ghee, or coconut oil. Same prep period, same simple recipe -- only a slightly different feel and cook some time.

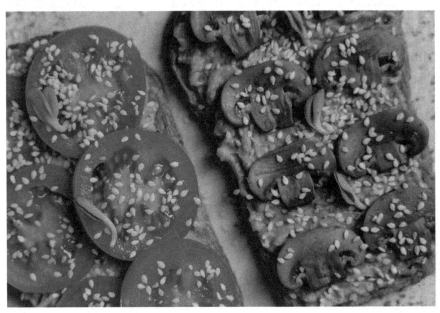

25. Simple Keto Bread

Just one slice of bread contains 15g of carbohydrates and virtually no fiber. Even whole wheat bread, though it contains more fiber and protein, is composed of 67% carbohydrate. About the ketogenic diet, carbohydrates generally only constitute 5-10percent of total calories. For many individuals, that is around 20-50 g every day. Fat and protein must constitute 70-80% and 20-25percent of total calories.

To put it differently, just one sandwich -- With just two bits of white bread will wipe out your whole carbohydrate intake daily. If you are trying to maintain your carbohydrate count low, routine store-bought bread is out of this question. Yet, with other fermented flours such as coconut almond and wheat flour getting increasingly more famous, there are loads of low carb bread recipes out there.

This keto bread is low carb and Packed with healthful fats. With only 5 grams net carbohydrates per piece, seven ingredients and 7 g of protein, then this recipe may satisfy any carbohydrate cravings while still keeping you into ketosis.

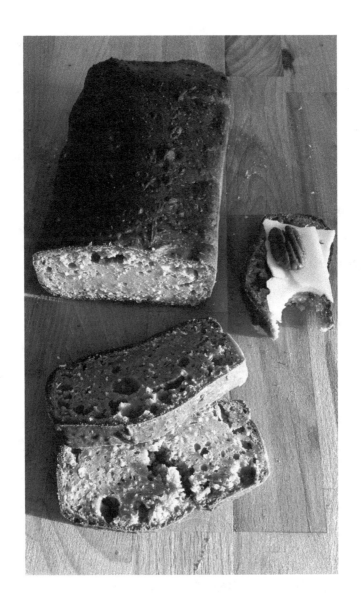

26. Keto Almond Bread

This keto almond bread comprises Less than 3 grams of carbs per piece and fits perfectly in your low carb meal program. It is packed with healthful fats, vitamins, minerals, and minerals such as vitamin E, riboflavin, manganese, magnesium, calcium, phosphorus, and iron. So, what is in this recipe which makes this sweet bread low-fat while still being a totally satiating beverage?

Ingredients

- 1/2 cup butter
- 2 Tbsp coconut oil
- 7 eggs
- 2 cups almond milk

Directions

- Preheat the oven to 355°F.
- Line a loaf pan with parchment paper.
- Mix the eggs in a bowl on top for as much as a couple of minutes.
- Add the almond milk, melted olive oil and melted butter into the egg whites. Continue to blend.
- Scrape the mixture to the loaf pan.
- Bake until a toothpick comes out clean.

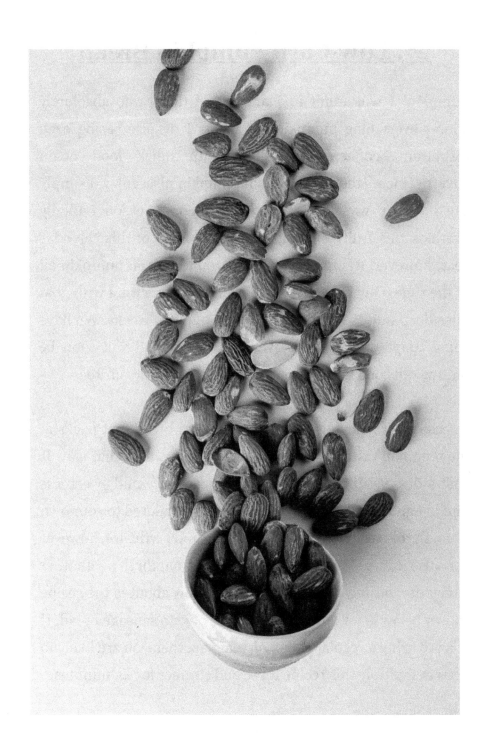

27. Low-Carb Pumpkin Bread

Pumpkin! I will admit it, I am one of those who absolutely adores everything pumpkin. As far as I despise seeing each restaurant, coffee shop, along with quick food chain advertisements their most recent pumpkin pleasantry, I simply can not help myself. It is too great! For a reason I totally overlook this fruit? For another two months of this calendar year, however, when autumn rolls around it is all pumpkin all of the time. Obviously, we have been experimenting with goat bites deep into the night for the last couple of weeks. We have got a couple that we have finalized today and will soon be putting out soon, but this one could just be my favourite.

In case you're looking for a keto pumpkin bread that packs at the pumpkin taste whilst not being too sweet then that is it! It isn't a dessert. It is comparable in consistency and sweetness into banana bread. The sweetness could be tailored to your own taste. In this recipe we use liquid stevia and erythritol, however you also can get by using only one or another, or another sweetener entirely. Another factor to know about is the recipe shown below is for 2 miniature loaves of keto sausage bread. If you are using a regular 8×4 inch loaf pan, then you are likely to need to multiply this recipe three and simmer for 45 minutes.

This recipe is as straightforward as it gets. You just blend everything into a food processor or with a hand mixer and then inhale it. Another neat thing about this recipe is the foundation can be substituted to accommodate virtually any taste that you need to attain, it does not need to be more pumpkin (but I am making the most of my three weeks of pumpkin this season). We have completed a lot of different breads utilizing this foundation. Most recently, we left a great loaf of cheddar chorizo bread.

Ingredients:
- 2 large eggs
- 1/2 cup Almond Flour
- 3 tablespoon 100% pumpkin puree
- 1/2 tsp Pumpkin Pie Spice
- 1 tablespoon erythritol Optional
- 1/4 tsp vanilla extract
- 2 tablespoon Butter melted
- 15 Drops Liquid Stevia Could be subbed for different sweeteners
- 1/4 tsp Pink Himalayan Salt
- 3 tablespoon walnuts

Directions:
- Preheat oven to 350 degrees.

- Blend all ingredients aside from the walnuts into a bowl. Mix with a hand mixer using a food processor.
- Insert 2/3 of those walnuts and gently mix with a spatula.
- Pour the mix into the miniature loaf pans. If you would like to utilize a regular 8 x 4 inch loaf pan, then multiply this recipe by 3 occasions.
- Top with the rest of the walnuts. Bake for half an hour in 350 degrees.
- Remove from oven and let it cool for 10 minutes. Enjoy.

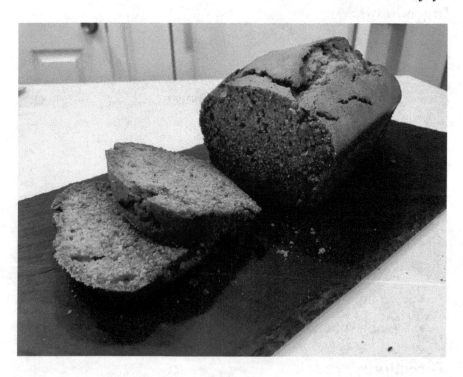

28. Keto Cheesecake

Since most cheesecakes are Flourless, changing the recipe to become keto friendly does not need many adjustments in any way. I began with my preferred go-to coriander and just altered three items: the thickener, the sweetener, along with the crust.

This keto cheesecake crust requires Almond milk as the foundation -- in case you do not have some available, just slip raw almonds or pecans in a food processor till they turn into some flour consistency. Or you could use another crust recipe or perhaps produce the cheesecake crust less in case you would rather, and every slice is going to have only 200 calories and below two grams of net carbohydrates.

You can use your preferred sweetener, Like erythritol or xylitol for glucose free. Normal sugar, maple sugar, and coconut sugar additionally all function in the recipe (it will not be ketogenic but may nevertheless consume much less sugar and fewer calories compared to conventional cheesecakes, whilst tasting equally as yummy).

Baking Tips for Your Very Best Cheesecake

The Main thing with Cheesecakes is not to overbeat the batter, which might introduce air bubbles which may burst from the oven and lead to cracking.

Similarly, permitting the cheesecake cool Gradually prevents any sudden temperature fluctuations which could also lead to the cake to decode.

No water tub is demanded; however, I really do Prefer to set a skillet with water beneath the cheesecake since it cooks, that adds warmth into the oven and also behaves as a further buffer against the notorious cheesecake cracking. If you would like to bypass the bowl of water, or even in case your cheesecake does wind up breaking for almost virtually any reason, all isn't lost: it is easy to conceal the cracks using a coating of fresh berries, whipped cream, or maybe even some healthful.

Ingredients
- 24 ounce cream rice or cheese lotion cheese
- 2 cups yoghurt, for example as coconut milk yogurt
- 2 1/2 teaspoon pure vanilla extract
- 1 tablespoon lemon juice, optional
- 2/3 cup erythritol (sugar maple Syrup also do the job for non-keto)
- 1/4 cup almond milk

Directions

Don't hesitate to utilize a store-bought crust or create this crust less, or this is your crust I've used: two cups vanilla or pecan bread (it's possible to combine nuts in a food processor to generate pasta), 1/4 teaspoon salt, and 4-6 tbsp roasted coconut oil OR sufficient water to make it a bit tacky. Blend all the ingredients, pour into a lined 8 or 9-inch springform pan, then press down equally, then put aside while you make the filling.

Preheat oven to 350 F. Fill any skillet about halfway up with water and put it at the oven's reduced rack. Bring cream cheese at room temperature and then beat all ingredients in a blender. I do typically incorporate the lemon to get a timeless cheesecake taste, but it is going to still work for those who do not have some available and will need to leave it all out. Spread filling on top of prepared crust. Set on the center rack (over the rack together with all the water bowl). Bake 30 minutes (or even 38 minutes when with an 8-inch pan), and don't open the oven whatsoever during that time. When time is up, nevertheless don't start the oven, however switch off the heat and allow the cheesecake sit in the oven an extra five minutes. Then remove from the oven, it will nonetheless seem underdone. Let cool in the counter 20 minutes, then wash immediately, during which time it will firm up greatly. As I mention at the article, the heating times are significant so that the cake melts slowly and consequently doesn't crack. Store leftovers covered in the fridge 3-4 times, or slit and freeze if wanted.

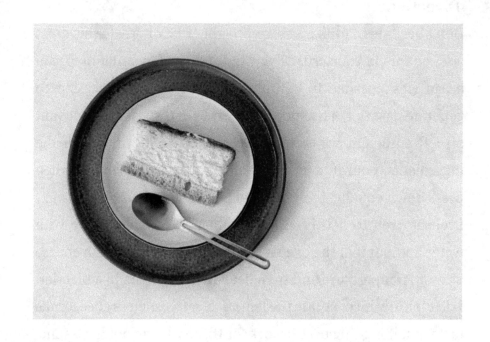

29. Keto Brownies

Rather than regular bread, these Brownies utilize fine almond meal or almond milk (ground-up almonds), which makes them equally flourless and gluten free of charge.

If you can discover Dutch cocoa powder I Highly advise using it when called for, since that is the sort of cocoa generally utilized in boxed brownie mixes, therefore it is what's going to make them flavor the most genuine.

Most frequent grocery shops should Market it look for the phrases "processed with alkali" on the area listing, and that is the kind to use. (Routine unsweetened cocoa powder needs to be used for your first 1/4 cup at the recipe)

The yellow chocolate brownies could be Made with regular glucose (such as non-keto) or granulated erythritol. When making them keto, then make certain to purchase granulated erythritol, not roasted. Or to get paleo brownies, then you might even use sugar.

While I haven't tried the recipe Allulose or stevia, don't hesitate to experiment using a granulated stevia mix if you desire, and make sure you report back to different subscribers should you.

Ingredients

- 1 cup good almond flour
- 1/4 cup cocoa powder
- 2 tablespoon Dutch cocoa or extra Normal
- 1 teaspoon baking powder
- 1/2 teaspoon salt
- 1/3 cup melted coconut butter or oil
- 3 tablespoons water or extra oil
- 2 eggs2 or two flax eggs
- 2/3 cup granulated erythritol or Normal sugar
- 1 teaspoon pure vanilla extrac.

Directions

- Preheat the oven at exactly 350 F. Grease an 8-inch pan, or line with parchment. Mix all ingredients well. Distribute evenly into the pan. Smooth down, utilizing another sheet of parchment if necessary. Bake 20 minutes to the middle rack, and then let cool completely and they'll continue to business. Additionally, they firm up much more should you refrigerate quite professionally covered overnight.

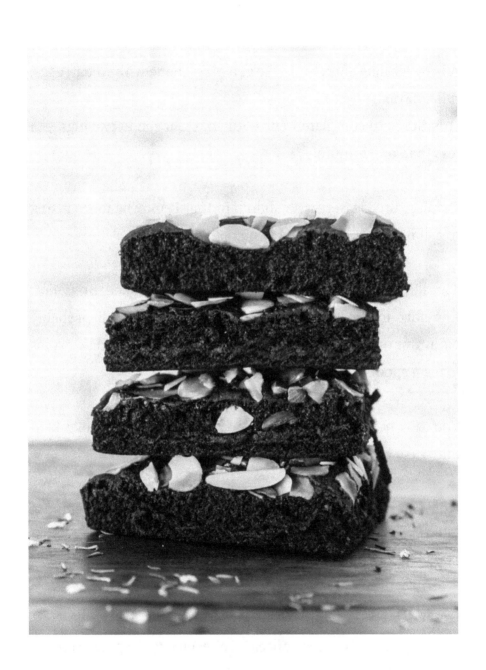

30. Keto Mug Cake

A brownie-like chocolate cake at a Mug, made with wheat, eggs, milk, or oil.
It Is Going to completely solve All your Chocolate cravings... in less than one minute!

Frankly, this dessert is so abundant that It may be more fitting to call it a chocolate cup brownie in lieu of a cake.

The flavor reminds me of this Ultimate Unbaked Brownies, therefore in case you enjoy that recipe, then you'll probably enjoy this one also -- it is like eating a heap of unbaked brownies using a spoon!

You can opt to use vanilla or nuts Flour with this particular keto mug cake free of egg, whatever's easier.

I have recorded the 3 variants Below that I have attempted (almonds, pecans, and vanilla milk), however I bet other people might get the job done also.

Ingredients

- 1/3 cup almonds or pecans, or even 6 tablespoon Almond milk (nut-free variant here)

- 1 tablespoon + 2 tsp ginger powder
- 1 tablespoon granulated erythritol or glucose or sweetener of choice
- Pinch stevia, or extra 2 tsp sugar
- 1/8 teaspoon salt
- 1/4 teaspoon baking powder
- 3 tablespoons milk of selection, or two if using Liquid sweetener
- 1/4 teaspoon pure vanilla extract
- Optional chocolate chips or glucose Free chocolate chips

Directions

- If using almonds, then grind them into a blender or food processor to attain a flour-like consistency. It'll be coarser than should you use almond milk (hence the vanilla bits it is possible to see in the photographs), but the two versions do the job.
- Blend all ingredients in a greased ramekin or little mug. You can preheat your oven at 350F for approximately ten minutes, or cook in microwave. If microwaving, timing will fluctuate based on wattage and desirable gooeyness. I began using 30 minutes, then additional two 15-second periods then. The cake will probably seem somewhat gooey once it comes out, and it firms up as it warms. But

there is no need to wait around for it to firm up a lot of - - this dessert is intended to be eaten directly from the mug!

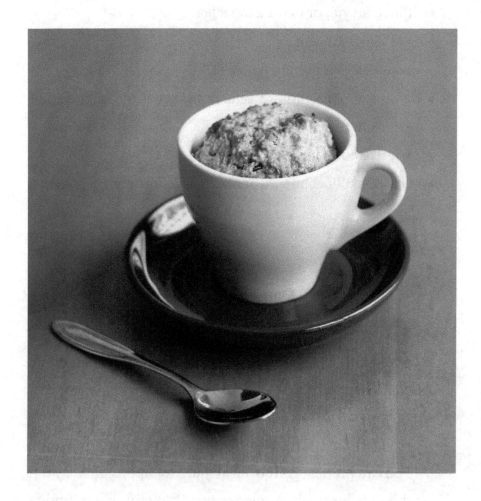

Why the Ketogenic Diet Impacts Fat Burn?

Keto helps you eliminate weight and Make some positive changes to your own life. The high fat, low-carb diet also has gained a great deal of popularity in the past several decades, making a whole neighborhood of keto-praising eaters.

Contrary to sugar restriction, keto Helps you eliminate weight by placing your body into ketosis. When you consume minimal carbs, your body produces ketones for energy. Ketones are created on your liver from fatty acids present in your body fat. Thus, your liver really burns fat to produce ketones. Ketones are utilized for energy instead of carbohydrates.

As your system burns off fat as a Gas supply, you will begin to eliminate weight. You could be thinking about if keto can target particular problem areas, for example stomach fat. Losing abdomen fat is high on the priority list for lots of men and women. The fat on your stomach is visceral fat, and this can be a harmful kind of fat which resides deep within the stomach, encasing your inner organs. Visceral fat is related to cardiovascular disease and type two diabetes.

Technically, you cannot spot-target Fat areas such as reduction. Your entire body determines where weight reduction will happen. But, keto could possibly be practical for removing stubborn belly fat.

Belly fat, or visceral fat, also stems from a mix of enzymes along with a diet high in refined carbohydrates and sugar. Visceral fat could quickly become inflamed, which makes it extremely stubborn to shed and harmful to surrounding arteries. A well-formulated keto program has powerful anti-inflammatory consequences, which makes it a lot easier to shed excess belly fat.

Keto alone probably Won't be enough to eliminate a lot of fat. Keto works well together with high-intensity interval training (HIIT) exercises). Speak with your physician prior to starting any new diet or exercise program.

Common Queries About Keto

Should I attempt keto, does this mean that I could Never eat carbs?

No. But You'll Need to Significantly cut down your carbohydrate intake in the beginning. Following two to three weeks, you'll have carbohydrates on particular events --so long as you come back to the diet shortly after.

Can I lose muscle mass?

There's some danger of losing weight Mass in almost any diet program. But, higher protein consumption and ketone levels may diminish muscle loss, especially if you power train.

Imagine if I'm always fatigued?

If you are always feeling exhausted or Fatigued, you might not be in complete ketosis. Your body may not be utilizing ketones and fats at the utmost truly effective way. You ought to try reducing your carbohydrate intake or adding supplements to your daily diet. MCT oil or exogenous ketones will help combat fatigue.

I've digestion difficulties. What if I really do?

Digestive disturbances are a very standard Side impact of changing to a ketogenic diet. Symptoms ought to pass in a few weeks. Meanwhile, consider eating more high-fiber veggies or supplementing with calcium to ease constipation.

How to Gain Energy with Keto

The Way to High-Carb Diet Makes You Allergic

From the Standard American Diet (SAD), Carbohydrates are king.

If a meal does not begin with a Vitamin foundation (think: rice or pasta), it generally has them onto both sides (i.e., mashed potatoes, corn or beans).

The Issue is a higher intake of the Macronutrient can be damaging to your vitality levels.

See, if you eat carbohydrates, the starches Found in these are converted into simple sugar levels, or sugar.

Your own body then absorbs the sugar Also gives you an energy boost.

However, in order to do this, it requires Insulin, which is produced from the pancreas, to transfer that sugar from the blood to your own cells to utilize them.

So, because your blood sugar levels rise Post-tacos, insulin has been released to assist carry this fresh influx of energy into significant cells inside the body.

This procedure also helps decrease your Blood sugar levels back to normal.

Once your body gets sufficient, it will Send a sign to a liver and muscle cells to keep the excess energy, or sugar, for afterwards. Insulin also sends a different signal into a liver allowing it understand your sugar stores are now complete.

However, that is only if all goes well. In case you have insulin resistance or decreased insulin sensitivity, then your entire body struggles to consume this energy.

Additionally, it has Difficulty handling Insulin correctly and ends up having it to find the business completed and usher those sugar molecules in cells. Your pancreas senses that this issue and makes a spike of insulin to attempt and keep up with the requirements and level out your glucose.

Even still, it is not always sufficient to Handle the job. Sometimes you are left with excess sugar in your blood.

When This Occurs, you encounter a Massive surge in power immediately, but it is quickly followed with a major fall from the contrary direction.

You are left feeling lethargic and Craving additional energy in the shape of sugar and carbohydrates.

And you do not Have to Have insulin Resistance (IR) for it to take place. In my instance I believed every bit of this insulin spike once I ate, however, after several tests was not believed insulin resistant.

So, because I kept undergoing these Crazy highs and lows through the day, and I felt hungry and tired, I chose to perform a small experimentation:

I tapered my carbohydrates and additional healthful Fats in their location simply to find out how things might change. And they certainly did.

I noticed that a drastic improvement in my Energy degrees and that I experienced daily energy slumps which created it impossible to focus and complete my job later daily.

I don't used to bite 24/7 either.

And I'd continued energy rather than Being strapped to the carb-powered energy roller coaster I had been used to.

So why and how does this basic Switch from carbohydrates to fat supply you extra energy?

The Science Behind the Best Way to Ketogenic Diet Enhances Energy

Together with the regular SAD, your system is Educated to operate on carbohydrates.

It becomes the main fuel supply and you are feeling tired and lethargic till you receive the next spoonful of carbohydrates (aka sugar).

This manner of eating generates a vicious Cycle that may result in overeating, low power and storage.

You will confront zero of those issues on a ketogenic diet.

Rather than fueling with carbohydrates, you will Be draining your entire body of its own surplus shops and depriving it with healthful fats.

The average man about the SAD eats Around 225 g of carbohydrates daily. A keto diet restricts this to less than 50 g.

This forces the body to change to a "fat accommodated" condition where it depends on fat stores rather than carbohydrates for energy.

Your body will not shout at you for More energy; it may tap to its shops (your own fat) at any moment.

You will like a continuous, steady Flow of keto energy rather than drops through the day since you are not spiking your glucose.

Then you will be able to kiss these Afternoon energy slumps along with the dreaded hangries bothersome both your loved one's members and colleagues forth once and for all. However, for this glorious stage, you want to create the transition from relying upon carbohydrates for fuel to working on fat.

If you are thinking about a keto diet, then Have a look at this manual to begin on the ideal foot.

To give you a notion of what to anticipate, let us discuss exactly what exactly your energy levels will be like throughout your keto transition .

Everything You Can Expect During the Transition

Based on how carb-heavy your daily diet Was to start with, the transition into keto does not have to be difficult or it might be a small struggle, and this can certainly impact your energy levels.

If you are among those unlucky few, the transition can permit you to go through the keto influenza, a state that feels exactly like the usual influenza (believe: stomach pains, nausea, nausea, depression, brain fog, etc.).

This isn't the body's way of Creating the transition from utilizing carbohydrates for energy into Ketosis. In this time period, you might not believe your best and you also likely won't have a lot of energy. It is ideal to take it simple and go light on actions, both emotionally and emotionally, as you create the transition.

For many, this period can last one or Two times as many as many weeks. However, the very fact to remember is it's only momentary. When you make the change to ketosis, you will not encounter these signs or extreme fluctuations in energy levels. That said, the majority of men and women begin to observe a gap in their own energy levels right after they have left the transition. This usually means that you might begin to feel better over a couple of days or at about a couple of weeks. And, unlike most carb-induced energy spikes, then this brand new found energy will last to endure for so long as you remain in Ketosis. I really do have a word of warning for the fellow female subscribers, and that I will go over in another segment, about time their keto transition using their menstrual cycles.

Keto Energy and Female Hormones

If you are on your life span, your cycle may cause massive changes in your own energy levels.

At the first fourteen days and top up to childbirth, your estrogen levels are high, so you are going to have greater energy, an improved disposition, and also, for a few, you will also be outgoing. But after puberty strikes and you begin to input the next and fourth months of your cycle, then all bets are off.

Since your system falls in estrogen and Increases in fertility, your own energy levels generally have a nosedive.

There is more certainty to be Hungrier and crave carbohydrates and carbonated snacks in this period also.

This Is the Reason Why it's particularly important to your intake of protein and fat (just marginally here) to fight pesky carbohydrate cravings on the next and fourth week of the cycle.

But it's also a Fantastic idea to prevent Transitioning into a keto diet in this time, if at all possible.

As You're already low on electricity, it is not the cleverest to taxation your body farther by pushing to change energy sources concurrently also.

You are really better off Transitioning through the second or first week of the cycle by now your next week rolls around, you are going to have the continuing energy to make it through it without even having rapid carbohydrate snacks.

But if you Want a little Assistance, there is also one more key to creating the keto transition simpler: exogenous ketones.

Exogenous Ketones

Exogenous ketones are just one of these Products which appear too good to be true. Would you take a pill or a powder and also immediately get the advantages of ketosis?

Well, it is not that simple. But if you are considering the advantages of a ketogenic diet, exogenous ketones are certainly something to check into.

These nutritional supplements come in various types and you are able to use them for various functions, from diminishing keto influenza symptoms to improving physical and psychological performance.

Ketosis is a metabolic condition at which your body utilizes ketones (rather than sugar) for energy. Unlike what a lot of men and women presume, your body is able to run remarkably well without relying upon blood sugar or blood glucose.

You are at a state of ketosis when your own body is operating on energy generated by its ketones, however, you might also get there using exogenous ketones. Ketosis can result in a plethora of health benefits, from decreasing chronic inflammation into fat reduction and muscle building maintenance.

The ketones the own body makes are called endogenous ketones. The prefix "endo" signifies something is generated within your own body whereas the prefix "exo" means it is derived out of your own body (like in a nutritional supplement).

Low-Carb & Keto Snacks for Gas & Energy

When it comes to snacking a Ketogenic, low-carb, energy is of the nature. You would like fuel with only a few snacks. Obviously, the principal focus is fat. Oh, and obviously we need a scarcity of carbohydrates. You're able to throw a few proteins to the mixture if it is logical. Otherwise, there are only a few limitations in our manner. See, somebody on a standard diet may reach for a bit of fruit, a nip or a candy to get a bite, but there is a massive issue with this: that is not fuel. Your body is likely to burn through that sugar, and it is likely to be clever enough to desire more since you require constant energy consumption for constant energy output.

The keto diet speeches that issue by supplementing fat rather. It retains the flame for a good deal longer with a ton less tending to. These are a few yummy, high fat, low-fat snack selections that you on the move, when you have got the munchies, or else you only need a boost.

Some Keto Snacking Essentials:

- Fantastic excellent protein powder. Many keto biscuits and candies utilize protein powder to mass up the protein material, needless to say, include flavour, and inhale.

- Avocado. You are likely to locate avocado at a great deal of keto bite alternatives, whether it's obvious. Always have a couple handy.

- Unsweetened chocolate. If your snacks are inclined to be selected from the sweet tooth, you need that 100% -- the real thing!

- Coconut oil. Y 'understand... since coconut oil fixes almost everything. You likely have some. Otherwise, it is time to stock up.

- Swerve sweetener. Here is the preferred, wholesome, aspartame-free, natural sweetener for controlling the keto tooth. Get it, use it, enjoy it.

- Cheese. By itself or alone, fantastic quality cheese really is really a lifesaver when it comes to snacking and keto bite recipes. Maintain a variety.

Healthy Snack

Salad Sandwiches

Is not the best Aspect of this sandwich What is within the bread? Rather than swearing off sandwiches, then have a suggestion and get started utilizing huge leaves of lettuce, chard, or collards as leftovers to your favorite sandwich fillings. Seriously, if you're able to set it in a sandwich then you are able to set it to some low carb foliage. This cuts a few carbs from your bite, and in addition, it adds sugars.

Cheese Covered Grapes

Here Is a low-carb snack which will Look somewhat odd at first, but you may just get hooked on it. All these truffle-like snacks out of Healthful Pursuit really are a bit sweet and just a tiny bit sour. To create them, simply press a fresh grape to a chunk of your favorite goat cheese and then roll everything in certain chopped pistachios.

Pickled Avocado

We have done a Great Deal of things with Avocado, however till today, pickling was not among them. We all know we can only place some lettuce right to a vinegar-based mix to raise the avocado taste into cravable, snackable land. This bite demonstrates that avocados do not Require corn chips to Create an Amazing snack

Low-Carb Granola Bars

It's possible for you to take a lot of these Carbohydrates from your granola bars using seeds, nuts, and coconut scents to earn snackable low-fat bars which are just as pleasing as their counterparts that are humorous.

Cucumber Salad

The bite salad out of the Ketovangelist Kitchen is a lower carb eating savior. Smother celery and pineapple with fresh veggies to elevate the easy green veggies into gourmet land. This green mixture has lots of taste to wave you over to another meal, zero carbohydrates necessary.

Tofu Spread using Zucchini Slices

The foodie behind Vegetarian Gastronomy combines kale with garlic, oil, and ginger to produce a creamy spread that matches perfectly with an assortment of vegetables. Smear the carrot mix on new zucchini pieces to create a low-carb snack with all of the satisfying taste of a noodly lasagna.

Pecans

Having a rich, almost buttery taste, Low-carb pecans create a satisfying snack, if they are roasted, raw, or dusted with salt and fresh veggies. Pecans are packaged with good-for-you fats, including filling nourishment vitamin E.

Peanut Butter Balls

Peanut butter chunks will come into the Rescue any moment you encounter a costly snack attack. Made with only a couple of straightforward ingredients which are easy to keep available, the chunks do not even have to get cooked.

Pumpkin Butter Slice

It's two lovely layers for You eager for snack period. 1 layer incorporates rich and smooth pumpkin puree, strawberry seed butter, and pepitas. Another coating features foul-smelling chocolate and sweet vanilla taste. Healthy snacking hasn't looked really decadent.

Kale Chips

Why create chips from starchy Potatoes whenever there are all those amazing low-carb vegetables which crisp like magic? You may purchase premade kale chips in the supermarket (only check the tag for more sugars) or create your own in your home. Only toss lettuce leaves at a spoonful of olive oil along with your favorite toppings and bake at 350 degrees until crispy. Remember to eliminate the stalks; the rancid pops will prevent your chips out of crisping up.

CONCLUSIONS

Carbohydrates have been the Outcasts of this food world - delivered to the courageous step for endangering our waistlines. But they are crucial element of a balanced, healthful diet, critical for any variety of physiological processes to assist us daily.

So regardless of the low carb diet tendency Taking the findings published today verifying that low-fat diets aren't any more powerful than conventional low-carb diets, aren't any surprise. Carbs have been public enemy #1, particularly for those attempting to eliminate weight, but in precisely the exact same time, there is also a great deal of confusion about what they're.

No, milk products, such as butter, are believed fats. But carbohydrates are a far bigger food collection which goes beyond white bread as well as bread.

Today's fad, the keto diet concentrates on high fat, moderate protein and low carbohydrate targeted primarily in the fitness center and weight loss marketplace. It is predicting the keto diet since ketones will be the origin of energy the body uses if it is burning off fat.

In the Brief term, low carbohydrate Diets can be useful for weight reduction. On the other hand, the health consequences of keeping ketosis for lengthy intervals are unknown, particularly on the intestine microbiomes and ought to be supervised by a medical professional such as a dietitian. That said, I have seen a surge of "keto-friendly" goods from the mainstream marketplace over the previous two years such as the baking industry.

Most of Us know that sugar Is Vital For the sweet flavor. But sugar extends past sweetness and can be a significant component for purpose such as color, feel, and nourishment. While I state sugar, I am talking about table sugar (sucrose.) That makes it trickier to make a low-carb bread or baked great. I have seen a few baking disasters since the sugar from the recipe was meddled with. A couple baking organizations are especially focusing on the keto marketplace. Even substituting maple syrup or honey to table sugar generates new interactions which won't behave just like glucose, resulting in rather different results, like utilizing low sugar additives.

Making a shift isn't a simple job. In case you've tried it, you might have come across a few of the most frequent challenges, such as cravings, sluggishness, and brain fog. Additionally, it may be a psychological challenge; resulting in doubts and needs you didn't know where significant for you. However, you don't need to worry anymore! By introducing Keto bread in your diet plan, you can't just encourage your wellbeing and well-being, however, you might also ease in the lifestyle in a means that's less daunting and more prohibitive compared to other options until you.

The more you understand about the Keto diet Generally, the more you're able to know why Keto bread is still an organic food to Incorporate on your eating program. It Might Sound counter-intuitive to add bread into a low-carb eating strategy; nonetheless, Keto bread is very exceptional due to the Ingredients used in creating it. Some areas sell Keto bread baked for You, however, there are lots of unique recipes you may try out to include it in to Your own Keto plans. You Might Have heard people claiming it's "filthy Keto" into Include substitutions on your daily meal plan, for example bread, but as you Read the info presented within this audiobook you may learn not Just the reason it's helpful to incorporate it on your Keto diet plan, but also why it's necessary!

KETO BREAD COOKBOOK

THE ULTIMATE EASY LOW-CARB COOKBOOK WITH DELICIOUS BAKERY KETOGENIC RECIPES.

Dorothy Yosco

Bakery Ketogenic Recipes

Miss bread and other baked products on low carbohydrate or keto? It is quite feasible to create, but it needs different ingredients and it is only... different. Here is our guide to low-fat ingredients, significant things to think about and all our best low-carb recipes!

How Does it Work

Keto baking makes utilization of cereal flour replacements that could offer Building, binding influence and a few of the performance given by wheat germ proteins (e.g. gas retention, visco-elasticity). Substitutes contain floor forms/flour of:

Exotic fruits and tree nuts such as almonds, pecans, walnuts, hazelnuts, cashews, macadamia nuts, and pistachios (freezing of powerful flavours may be required)

Coconut

Flax meal (whole gold flax seed)

Sunflower and pumpkin seeds

Garbanzo beans, chickpeas, sesame seeds, soy milk (freezing of tastes may be required)

Protein isolates and protein targets on pulses and legumes

Gums like xanthan gum and CMC

Collagen

Eggs

Casein, cocoa powder, cheese, milk solids

Formulation

The next keto bread formulation utilizes no yeast. Additionally, it includes no or low levels of sugars and damaged carbohydrates and amylases. In cases like this, steam creation during baking in addition to chemical-leaveners are accountable for bread loaf increasing and quantity develop.

Keto Bread Formula

Ingredients for Low-Carb Baking

Low-carb baking differs from traditional baking. To start with you want to get to understand a lot of fresh ingredients utilized instead of bread made from wheat or other grains. The most usual ones we use in this book are vanilla flour, coconut milk and earth psyllium husk powder.

Almond flour1 is really a gluten free nut flour which should include nothing but earth blanched almonds. This usually means you could create your own in the home, away from scratch, by milling whole blanched almonds into a nice meal (unless you only wish to purchase it). Employing a spice or coffee grinder normally works best. Take care not to grind them too long or the nuts may discharge their fat and also you ´ll wind up with almond butter, that is a fantastic tasting nut butter although not exactly what you're going for when creating almond flour.

1 cup (240 ml) of wheat germ weighs 31/2 ounce. (99 g).

Coconut flour consists of Cold-pressed coconut flesh that has been dried and then ground into a nice meal. It's a feature coconut taste along with a high fiber material which contrasts the liquid within a dough. As it, such as almond milk, is fermented it will not create a soup increase like conventional pasta when yeast is included.

1 cup (240 ml) of coconut milk Weighs 41/2 ounce. (128 g).

Ground psyllium husk powder is 100 percent Pulverized psyllium husk cubes and can be utilized to provide a bread-like feel to what you are baking. As a result of the high fiber content it is frequently sold as a diuretic that could be useful to know in case you've got a sensitive digestive tract. When adding it into a liquid it becomes a gel-like material. It works somewhat like gluten in conventional baking, making it feasible to take care of the dough when forming or rolling it.

1 tbl of earth psyllium husk powder Weighs (10 g).

These products tend to disagree a Lot between various brands that makes low-fat baking somewhat catchy. By way of instance, some manufacturers of earth psyllium husk powder colour the bread purple. It does not appear to impact the flavor however, leaves the outcome somewhat longer... purple. The number of carbohydrates in coconut and almond flour may also change quite a difference between various brands. Read the labels and decide on the best one available.

Substituting flours

A frequent question is if you are able to Substitute almond milk for coconut milk as well as also the other way round. Yes, frequently you can although not in equal quantities. 1 cup of almond milk may be substituted for 1/3 cup of bread. 1/3 cup of coconut milk may be substituted for 2/3 cup almond milk + 1.5 tbsp of ground psyllium husk powder. The numbers might want to be corrected based upon what brands you are using.

Processing

Processing of keto bread can be very distinct from yeast-leavened bread created out of wheat-flour. The subsequent is a step by step keto baking process:

1. Ingredient scaling

2. Eggs prep and 1st blending. Separate the eggs and place the whites and cream of tartar in a large mixing bowl and blend on high speed till stiff peaks form.

3. 2nd Mixing. Mix egg yolk, almond Flour, butter, baking powder, salt, stevia, and 1/3 of those egg whites foam till a thick, uniform batter kinds.

4. Twist the foam. Fold in the rest Whipped egg whites in two parts.

5. Depositing or panning. Grease with Coconut oil spray before panning. An 8 x 4-inch loaf pan is generally utilized.

6. Baking. Given that the high density of this Formula, baking is performed in 400--420°F (204--216°C) into an internal temperature of 204°F (95°C). This typically requires 25--35 minutes. The more complicated the oven temperature, the longer the time.

7. Depanning

8. Cooling to loaf inner temperature of 95--105°F (35--40°C) prior packaging.

9. Packaging or functioning

Application
Keto baking is one form of fermented baking. This is because the majority of wheat germ substitutes and ingredients used in the creation of keto baked products come from fermented sources which don't belong to some Triticum species or alternative possibly gluten-containing cereals.

General guidelines:

- Mixing: it's essential to avoid any contamination of egg whites using butter since fat could create the egg to divide and reduce the capability to entrap atmosphere. Strict cleaning procedures such as gear, process tools and utensils must be carried out before beginning new batches.

- Baking: Vitamin profiling is a fantastic tool for controlling and monitoring the baking procedure. Given the radically different formulation in conventional bread, it's a good idea for optimum outcomes to comprehend the significance between oven ailments (timing/temperature) and microbial inactivation, crumb place and colour formation.

1. Keto "Rye" Bread

As you might have guessed, there's no Rye employed inside this bread - that I prevent using any kind of grains. Rather, this recipe depends on flax meal and coconut bread. I have never actually liked the flavor of the majority of flax breads, but that one tastes good! It made me realize just how small changes make a difference. It tastes good with sweet butter or cream cheese on the top and it is ideal when toasted or produced as "panini".

As you won't find any real "rye" Inside this knockoff bread recipe, then you'll crunch on exactly the identical hearty texture that is almost equal to the true thing -- minus the power wreck afterwards. Love this "rye" bread toasted or as a panini. And should you would rather sourdough over rye to your bread of choice, then take a look at the following recipe. This bread is obviously high in fat and low in carbohydrates, so for breakfast, so I included some healthful protein and created a fantastic tasting panini with lettuce & spring bread! Bear in mind, protein is obviously satisfying, therefore adding moderate quantities to your daily diet can allow you to stay sated.

In comparison to bread, it will always be a little moist. To take out the moisture, then it's possible to simply toast it. In the event the complete recipe is a lot for you, make half of the batch keep a few in your freezer.

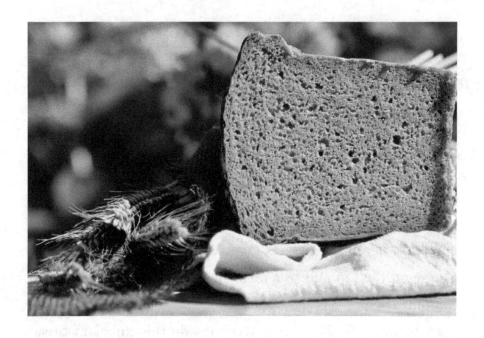

Ingredients

Dry Ingredients:

- 2 packed cups noodle meal (300 g/ 10.6 Ounce)
- 1 cup coconut milk (120 g/ 4.2 oz)
- 2 tablespoons caraway seeds (or lavender)
- 1 tablespoon + 1 teaspoon baking powder
- 1 tablespoon Erythritol or Swerve (10 grams / 0.4 ounce) or 3-5 drops liquid stevia
- 1/4 cup floor chia seeds (32 grams / 1.1 Ounce) or 1 teaspoon xanthan gum
- 1 tsp salt to taste (pink Himalayan rock salt)

Wet Ingredients:

- 8 eggs, divided
- 1/2 cup softened not melted ghee, 1/2 cup extra virgin olive oil (110 grams / 3.9 ounce)
- 2 tablespoon sesame oil, toasted
- 1/3 cup of apple cider vinegar (80 ml/ 2.7 fl oz)
- 1 cup hot water (240 ml/ 8 fl Oz)

Directions

- Transfer the oven rack into the middle place of the oven, and preheat to 190 °C/ / 375 °F (standard), or 170 °C/ / 340 °F (fan assisted). Add the dry ingredients into a large bowl and then completely whisk to blend (ground flaxseed, coconut milk, caraway, baking soda, Erythritol, salt and xanthan gum or floor chia seeds). It's particularly significant to evenly disperse the xanthan gum (or soil chia seeds).
- Separate the egg yolk from the egg whites and then maintain the egg whites apart. Add softened ghee or butter toasted sesame oil to the eggs. (Note: Though the

recipe does not request dividing the eggs, I discovered that doing this gets the bread fluffier.)

- Cream the egg yolk and also the ghee (butter or olive oil) until smooth. In another bowl, whisk the egg whites with cream of tartar till they produce soft peaks.
- Add your dry mix to the bowl together with the egg yolk mix and procedure nicely. It is a thick batter, also will come together gradually. Simply take some opportunity to be certain everything is completely blended.
- Add the vinegar and blend well.
- Add hot water and process until blended.
- Add the egg whites and fold in. Try not to deflate the batter entirely.
- Grease a big loaf pan with some ghee or butter and then put in the batter. Smooth out the batter evenly on the pan and then "cut" it on the top by means of a spatula to make a wave impact. Should you take advantage of a silicon loaf pan, then you won't have to wash it.
- Bake for about 50-60 minutes (depends on the oven). After the bread is ready, remove from pan to a cooling system, then let it cool completely.
- Slice thinly and enjoy!

2. Sourdough Keto Baguettes

Just because you are craving a pleasant Sub sandwich does not mean that you need to jump from ketosis to fulfill your taste buds.

With this low carb sourdough baguette Recipe, you are able to whip up and eat a sandwich how you truly want without destroying your hard work. This might help you package keto-friendly lunches for job also. Make the following keto bread recipe and you will also slip more micronutrients in daily.

Ingredients

Dry ingredients:
- 1 1/2 cup almond milk (150 grams / 5.3 Ounce)
- 2/3 cup psyllium husks - will probably be Powdered, can create about 1/3 cup psyllium husk powder (40 g/ 1.4 oz)
- 1/2 cup coconut milk (60 g/ 2.1 oz)
- 1/2 packaged cup noodle meal (75 grams / 2.6 Ounce)
- 1 teaspoon baking soda
- 1 teaspoon sea salt
-

Wet ingredients:

- 6 large egg whites
- 2 large eggs
- 3/4 cup low fat buttermilk (180 gram / 6.5 ounce) - full-fat could make them too thick and they may not grow
- 1/4 cup white wine vinegar apple Cider vinegar (60 ml/ 2 fl oz)
- 1 cup lukewarm water (240 ml/ 8 fl Ounce)

Directions

- Preheat the oven at exactly 180 °C/ / 355 °F (fan assisted), or 200 °C/ / 400 °F (standard). Utilize a kitchen scale to quantify all of the ingredients. Add all of the dry ingredients in a bowl (almond milk, coconut milk, ground flaxseed, psyllium powder, baking soda, and salt).
- In another bowl, combine the eggs, egg whites along with buttermilk.
- Add the egg mixture and then procedure well with a mixer till the dough is still thick. Add vinegar and warm water and process until well blended.
- Don't over-process the dough. With a spoon, then create 8 routine or 16 miniature baguettes and set them onto a baking tray lined with parchment paper or even a non

stick mat. They'll grow, so be certain that you leave some distance between them. Optionally, score the baguettes diagonally and create 3-4 cuts.

- Put in the oven and cook for 10 minutes. After that, decrease the temperature to 150 °C/ / 300 °F (fan assisted), or 170 °C/ / 340 °F (normal) and bake for another 30-45 minutes (little baguettes will require significantly less time to cook).

- Remove from the oven, then allow the tray cool and set the baguettes onto a stand to cool to room temperature. Store them at room temperature when you're planning to utilize them in another few days or store in the freezer up to 3 weeks.

- Enjoy like routine baguettes! To conserve time, combine all of the dry ingredients beforehand and store in a ziplock tote and put in a tag with the amount of ingredients. Once ready to be boiled, simply put in the wet ingredients.

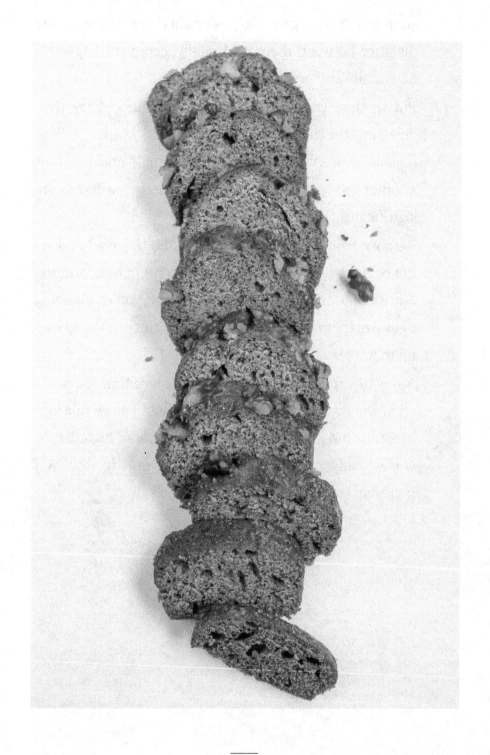

Keto Bread Troubleshooting

Lukewarm water in this recipe may Slow down the increasing impact of baking soda. I attempted both heated water and succulent and even though it made no real difference for baguettes, a few individuals have been suffering from air bubbles / hollow interiors after creating a loaf. More details about the best loaf are recorded here.

Ensure you utilize a kitchen scale to get Measuring all of the dry ingredients. Applying just cups might not be adequate to achieve best outcomes, particularly in baked products. Weights per cups and tablespoons can fluctuate based upon the product/brand or whenever you create you have ingredients (such as flax meal out of flaxseeds). Psyllium absorbs plenty of water. When baking using psyllium, you need to be sure to drink enough water during the day to stop constipation!

Use egg whites. The reason you Should not utilize just whole eggs is the bread would not rise with a lot of egg yolks inside. Do not squander them use them for creating Homemade Mayo, Easy Hollandaise Sauce or Lemon Curd. For precisely the identical reason, use low carb (not full-fat) buttermilk.

Eliminate moisture. Baked products that Utilize psyllium always end result is a bit moist feel. If necessary, cut on the baguettes in half and set into a toaster or in the oven prior to serving.

Don't use complete psyllium husks. Utilize a coffee grinder or a food processor to powder first.

I Don't recommend readymade psyllium husk powder. I have sliced dozens of keto breads also that I created them utilizing whole psyllium husks I roasted myself. Ready-made psyllium husk powder is frequently too delicate and leaves every keto bread overly dense, thick and flat. On occasion the bread would also receive a purple color and also an ammonia-like aftertaste (though that could possibly be associated with rancid carrot meal). Trust me, you do not need one of these in your bread! The very best approach to acquire the ideal flavor and texture is to purchase whole psyllium husks and powder in a coffee grinder using a food processor.

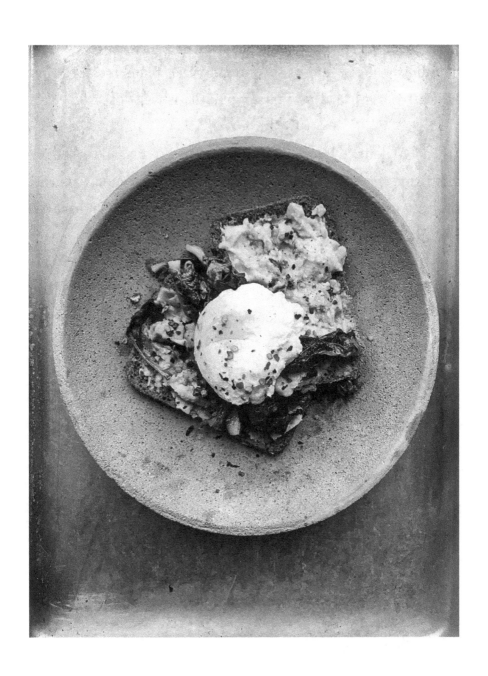

3. Low-Carb Cauliflower Bread

Cauliflower is the star of several keto Diet plans (such as this low carb berry bread). And its popularity is well deserved.

1 head of lettuce goes a very long way. It may be riced to substitute rice, so it could be turned into a crispy and flavorful cauliflower pizza crust, as well as baked in to cauliflower breadsticks.

It is Hard to locate low-carb bread Recipes that taste great, yet this berry bread is the exclusion. What is more, this recipe is not just simple -- it is also dairy-free and packed with protein and fiber. It genuinely imitates regular bread in texture and taste. You can add excitement to your soup with a few Italian spices to get a sweet treat or include a few drops and nut butter to get a fresh twist.

Salty or sweet, you will want to include This keto recipe for your low carb recipe listing.

This keto-friendly cauliflower bread Is:

- Comforting
- Delicious

- Warm

- Savory

- Paleo

- Dairy-free

The Key Ingredients are:

- Cauliflower florets

- Almond flour

- Eggs

- Psyllium husks

Optional additional ingredients:

- Sprinkle of salt

- Rosemary

- Oregano

- Black pepper

- Nut butter

- Parmesan cheese

Health Benefits of Cauliflower Bread

Cauliflower is among the very beloved vegetables in keto because of this. It is multipurpose, low carb, and packaged with macronutrients. It may surprise you to understand it may provide even more advantages in bread type.

1: **Could Enhance Your Digestion**

When it comes to gut digestion and health, fiber is the number one ally. Your body does not absorb and digest fiber at precisely the exact same manner it does with different carbohydrates. Rather, fiber pops around on your digestive tract, behaving as meals to your intestine bacteria and helping in bowel health in many of means.

This yummy cauliflower recipe includes 3.7 g of fiber in every piece, which not just lowers your internet carbohydrate intake but also keeps your digestion functioning smoothly and your intestine bugs contented.

Bulking and trimming your feces is Not the sole way fiber will be able to give you a hand. Getting your everyday dose may also help against lots of gastrointestinal disorders such as eczema, diverticulitis, hemorrhoids, along with duodenal cancer.

Nearly All the fiber from this Steak bread is arriving out of psyllium husk. Psyllium is a good source of soluble and insoluble fiber. If your uncertain of this gap, Here Is a small breakdown:

Soluble fiber: Slows down digestion. It creates a Gel on your intestines and may reduce cholesterol by binding to it on your digestive tract, and that reduces LDL on your blood.

Insoluble fiber: Reduce your own digestion. It adds Bulk to your stools also will aid their movement throughout your digestive Tract.

Psyllium husk Also Functions as a Prebiotic, which means that it feeds the good bacteria in the gut. Prebiotics assist your immune system by strengthening your shields against foreign germs and warding off problems such as diarrhea.

Psyllium husk Might Even be helpful in case You are fighting with inflammatory bowel problems. In a bunch of individuals with active Crohn's disease, the combination of psyllium and probiotics has been proven to be an effective treatment.

2: **Helps Protect Your Heart**

Fiber comes with a Fairly remarkable Effect On heart health too. In reality, the more fiber you consume, the not as likely you are to create high blood pressure, stroke, higher cholesterol, and CVD (cardiovascular disease.

Psyllium husk, in particular, includes Been analyzed as a source of fiber which can prevent CV. Cauliflower is loaded in a compound called sulforaphane. Sulforaphane is referred to as a direct antioxidant and might have heart-protective properties. 1 means that sulforaphane may safeguard your heart is via its capacity to improve specific antioxidant pathways, and that explains the reason why it's known as an "indirect antioxidant," an antioxidant.

If your heart stops becoming sufficient Blood -- and consequently oxygen there could be tissue damage, called ischemic injury. Fortunately, sulforaphane helps shield against irreparable harm and, thus, protects your listen. There is 1 hint to get the absolute most from cauliflower. It is possible to just release sulforaphane if you chop, slit, LOL, or chew over the cauliflower. It'd be reasonable to state that its heart-protective attributes are only waiting for one to trigger them.

Cauliflower is also an Excellent source of Vitamin C and vitamin folate. Studies have revealed that lack of these nutrients may be correlated with greater odds of developing cardiovascular disorders. Vitamin C is also critical for the optimum function of our immune system, whereas folate can help prevent certain Kinds of cancer like pancreatic and esophageal cancer

This exceptionally versatile veggie is Additionally a potassium powerhouse. Various studies have revealed that healthy intakes of the nutrient reveal a correlation with reduced blood pressure levels, which consequently reduces the chance of coronary heart disease.

May Promote Weight Loss

Several factors come into play You are attempting to shed weight. Obviously, exercise and picking the ideal foods ought to be on very top of your listing, but feeling and satisfaction complete also play a significant function.

The fiber from almond milk and Psyllium husk makes it possible to feel full and happy since it adds mass and slows digestion. And individuals who eat more fiber are inclined to be slimmer than people who prevent it.

Studies Also Have revealed that if You are obese and wanting to eliminate some unwanted pounds, including fiber to your daily diet can significantly improve weight reduction.

Ingredients

- 2 cups almond milk
- 5 eggs
- 1/4 cup psyllium husk
- 1 cup Milk rice

Directions

- Preheat oven to 350 °F.
- Line a loaf pan together with parchment paper or coconut oil cooking spray. Put aside.
- In a big bowl or food processor, combine the almond milk and psyllium husk.
- Beat in the eggs for as much as a couple of minutes.
- Mix from the pumpkin rice and combine well.
- Pour the pumpkin mixture to the loaf pan.
- Bake for up to 55 minutes.

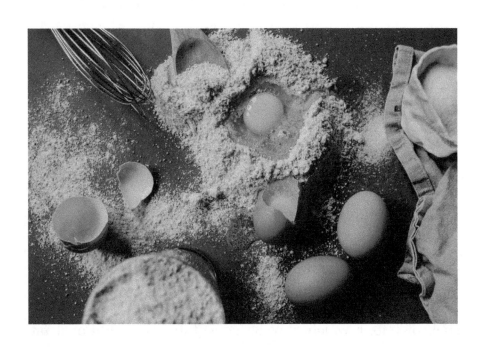

4. Rosemary and Garlic Coconut Flour Bread

How to Make It

After baking bread on a keto diet Have two choices of flours. Coconut almond and wheat milk. If you wish to try out a keto bread recipe with coconut milk then devote our additional recipe a go. Employing coconut milk causes a decrease calorie, flakier bread, and this is unquestionably a favorite around our property.

Insert a Lot of Fat

Fat is obviously your buddy on a Ketogenic diet plan and this particular bread recipe is no exception. This recipe requires a stick of butter which may be substituted for additional fat sources such as coconut oil, however, the wager results will include utilizing butter.

Usage Herbs and Spices

We use garlic and rosemary in this Recipe, but use whatever herbs and spices you would like. It's possible to exit the batter but keto breads tend to desire a little additional taste to enhance the flavor. Normal bread gets the yeast taste that is forfeited from low carbohydrates.

No Eggy Taste

This coconut chili bread doesn't Have the powerful egg flavor that lots of keto breads possess. It's a gentle coconut Flavor, with a rosemary and garlic coming. Should you still need less of an egg flavor, a surefire method to accomplish this is by including a very small splash of vinegar. Approximately 1 teaspoon is going to do.

Permit to Cool Before Slicing

This is essential! If you try cutting to this particular coconut flour loaf until it has chilled completely you are likely to wind up getting a crumbly mess. Coconut flour is exceptionally crumbly, and that means you are going to need to slice this using a cookie cutter in case you have one lying about. It takes approximately 60 minutes for this particular loaf to cool fully.

Store in the Fridge

This coconut milk bread, also only About all very low carb breads will need to be kept in the refrigerator. They'll go bad in a matter of days when kept on the counter because of their high moisture content. Pop up this in the refrigerator for around a week or two at the freezer it will last 1-2 weeks. I would rather slice the bread before freezing it.

Baking with Coconut Flour

Coconut flour is the favorite flour for quite a few reasons:
 Low Price
Gluten free
Excellent taste
You use less recipe
Our favorite brands to Search for are Anthony's or Bob's Red Mill.

Coconut Flour vs Almond Flour

A couple of things to remember when baking with coconut milk is it is quite tricky to substitute with wheat flour. You are better off looking a coconut milk recipe than attempting to convert one which utilizes almond flour. The cause of this can be coconut milk is significantly more resistant to fluids. So, where you'd require a couple cups of almond milk, you might just require half a cup of coconut milk.

How to Generate Coconut Flour Bread Boost

The unhappy fact is that coconut milk Bread won't rise. I am aware that it's unfortunate, however, two items are expected to earn bread rise. Gluten and yeast. You may earn a fantastic low-carb bread recipe which will grow, but it would not be gluten free. We mostly prefer to adhere with gluten free bread round the home.

Ingredients:

- 1/2 cup Coconut flour
- 1 stick butter (8 tablespoons)
- 6 large eggs
- 1 teaspoon Baking powder
- 2 tsp Dried Rosemary
- 1/2-1 teaspoon garlic powder
- 1/2 teaspoon Onion powder
- 1/4 tsp Pink Himalayan Salt

Directions
- Blend dry ingredients (coconut milk, baking powder, garlic, onion, rosemary and salt) into a bowl and put aside.

- Add 6 eggs into another bowl and beat with a hand mixer till you get view bubbles on very top.

- Melt the stick of the butter in your microwave and then gradually add it to your eggs because you conquer together with the mixer.

- Once dry and wet ingredients are fully blended in different bowls, gradually add the dry ingredients into the wet ingredients because you blend together with the hand mix.

- Grease an 8x4 loaf pan and then pour the mix to it evenly.

- Bake at 350 for about 40-50 minutes (time will be different based upon your oven).

- Permit it cool for 10 minutes before removing from the pan. Slice up and love butter or toasted!

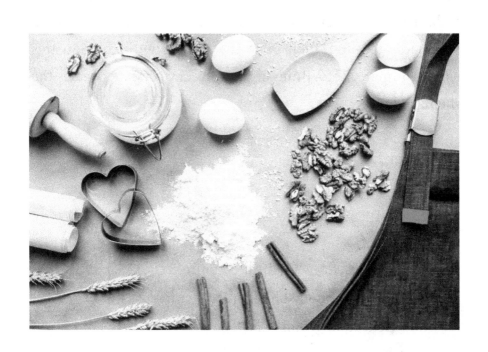

5. Keto Garlic Bread

This garlic keto bread would be the ideal Celebration appetizer appropriate for those after a healthier ketogenic strategy. It is diet-friendly and will not spike your blood glucose.

The two baguettes and chemical butter can be ready beforehand and crisped in under 15 minutes. If you cannot eat milk, forget the cheese topping, then swap the sourdough keto baguettes using Ultimate Keto Buns and apply lard or fat to earn the chemical butter.

Ingredients

Herb Compound Butter & Garlic:

- 1/2 cup of softened unsalted butter (113 G / 4 ounce)
- 1/2 teaspoon salt (I like pink lavender Salt)
- 1/4 teaspoon ground black pepper
- 2 tspn extra virgin olive oil (30 ml)
- 4 cloves garlic, crushed
- 2 tablespoon freshly chopped coriander or two Tsp dried parsley

Topping:

- 1/2 cup of grated Parmesan cheese (45 grams / 1.6 ounce)
- 2 tablespoons fresh parsley

Optional: garnish with additional virgin Olive oil

Option alternatives:

Ultimate Keto Buns
Nut-Free Keto Buns
Psyllium-Free Keto Buns
Flax-Free Keto Bread
Try unique tastes of keto Chemical butter
Rather than parmesan, attempt with cheddar, Manchego, Gruyere, or gouda.

Directions

- Ready the keto sourdough baguettes by obeying this particular recipe (you are able to create 8 routine or 16 miniature baguettes).
- Get the garlic butter (or some additional unsalted butter). Be certain all the ingredients have reached room temperature prior to blending them in a bowl.

- Cut the baked baguettes in half and then distribute the unsalted butter on top of every half (1-2 tsp per slice).
- Sprinkle with grated Parmesan and put back into the oven to clear up for a couple more minutes.
- Once completed, Evacuate from the oven.

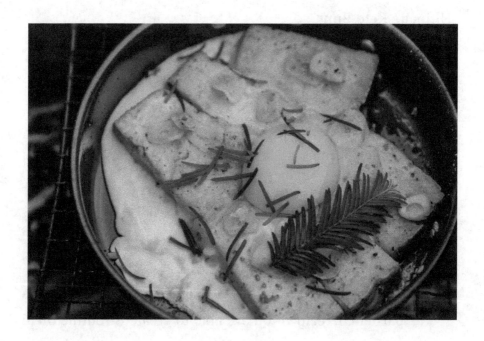

6. Cheesy Garlic Keto Breadsticks (2 Ways)

When beginning a new diet, then moving out to consume can end up being a struggle for numerous explanations. A few of the reasons people may find eating to be this hard is due to the deficiency of management and the numerous temptations they're faced with.

Most of Us know the sensation of sitting the table at the restaurant along with your own server systems you with a spoonful basket of hot breadsticks in his or her own hand. Together with all these Keto Breadsticks, you are going to have the ability to prepare yourself with no fear or anxiety about going on your keto macro objectives.

Making up just five grams of internet carbohydrates to get a serving of 2 breadsticks, you're still able to appreciate this satisfying fighter with no stress of being pumped out of ketosis. What exactly constitutes the ingredients in these very low carb breadsticks? A number of the vital elements include vanilla meal, coconut bread, shredded mozzarella cheese, greens and olive oil (or butter) olive oil, and also some other extra spices or herbs of your choice. What most individuals don't understand (and the number of people beginning the keto diet have begun to work out) is that mozzarella cheese leaves a wonderful low-carb curry base for several baking soda. The principal advantages of mozzarella cheese stem out of the abundance of minerals and vitamins. Mozzarella cheese is really a powerful supply of fat-soluble vitamins such as vitamin A, vitamin D, and vitamin E. It is also full of vitamin B6, biotin, thiamin, niacin, riboflavin, also naturally -- calcium.

These yummy keto breadsticks will be the Ultimate low-carb substitute for your favorite appetizer, packaging all of the wholesome fats with no abundant carbohydrates.

Ingredients

- 1 cup almond meal (or nut bread blend)
- 1 tbsp coconut flour
- 1/2 tbsp baking powder

- 1/2 tsp salt
- 1 1/2 teaspoons granulated garlic
- 2 cups shredded mozzarella
- 2 large eggs
- 1/4 cup jojoba oil melted grass-fed butter
- 1 tbsp Italian herb mix
- 1/4 cup shredded asiago or parmesan cheese
- 1 tbsp olive oil

Directions

- Pre-heat the oven to 400F.
- Put in a large bowl whisk together with the flour, baking powder, 1 tsp granulated salt and garlic.
- In a tiny, microwave-safe bowl, melt down the mozzarella. Microwave on high for 60-90 minutes.
- Whisk the eggs and coconut oil to the flour mixture, then fold into the melted mozzarella.
- Work fast while it is still hot.
- Flatten the dough on a 9" cast-iron or non skillet.
- Sprinkle with herb combination, asiago and olive oil. Bake for 10-15 minutes, until the cheese at the top is toasty.

- Remove from the oven and let it cool for 10 minutes. Then move the flatbread on a cutting board and cut to 10 sticks.

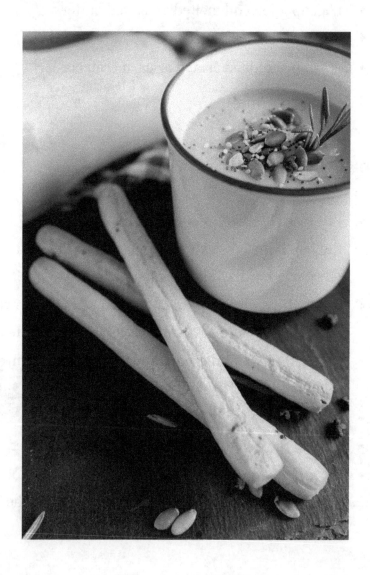

7. Keto Jalapeno Cheese Bread

This keto jalapeño bread is reminiscent of pizza! Merely requiring a single bowl that is a simple low-fat, nut-free bread choice to whip for sandwiches, a bite, or only a side.

Do not like jalapeños or creating this for those kiddos? Just leave off the jalapeños or swap them to get pepperoni or some other pizza fashion topping of your choice. This bread can be amazing if dunked into a little marinara or ranch dressing table.

Ingredients (makes 8 servings)

- 4 large eggs
- 2 tablespoons tbsp full-fat Greek yogurt (60 g/ 2.1 oz)
- 1/3 cup coconut milk (40 g/ 1.4 oz)
- 2 tablespoon whole psyllium husks (8 g/ 0.3 Ounce)
- 1/2 teaspoon sea salt
- 1 teaspoon fermented baking powder
- 1/2 cup shredded sharp cheddar Cheese, split (57 grams / 2 ounce)
- 1/4 cup of diced pickled jalapeños (28 G / 1 ounce)
- Couple chopped jalapeños for topping (14 G / 0.5 ounce)

Optional: serve with homemade Marinara Sauce or Ranch Dressing

Directions

- Preheat the oven at exactly 190 °C, or 170 °C/ / 340 °F (fan assisted) plus a baking sheet together with parchment paper. In a moderate bowl whisk together with the eggs along with Greek yogurt.
- Add coconut milk, psyllium husks, salt and baking powder.
- After easy stir in half the shredded cheddar cheese.
- Add the diced jalapeños.
- Press the dough to a 2.5 cm/ 1 inch thick ball onto the baking sheet. Top with remaining cheese and extra jalapeños if wanted.
- Bake for 15 minutes or till fluffy and golden. Cut into 8 squares.
- Serve hot or allow it to cool.
- Store in an airtight compartment in the refrigerator for about seven days.

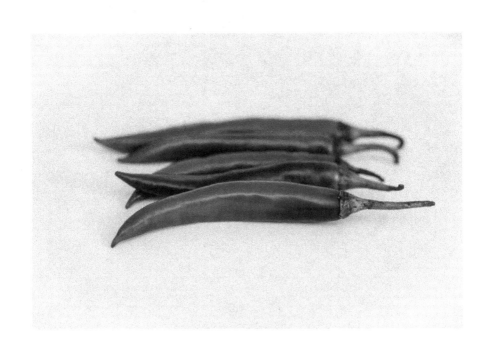

8. Low-Carb Spinach Dip Stuffed Bread

Jump the Terrible high-carb tortilla Chips which break when you dip them and attempt this packed poultry dip "bread" recipe which combines the very best of both worlds. In just 45 minutes, then you will have a dish guaranteed to be a hit regardless of who has to split a chunk off. And that also occurs with another recipe. The trickiest aspect of creating this really is forming the dough. I had a springform pan with it for advantage. The separate base makes it a whole lot simpler to form the dough, and then you'll be able to pop up the ring back after forming baking and storage. You might even utilize any other curved dish or perhaps merely a baking sheet lined with parchment paper.

Ingredients

"Bread" Dough

- 5 oz shredded mozzarella
- 1 oz shredded cheddar
- 1 oz cream cheese
- 1 tbsp butter

- 1/2 tsp Italian seasoning
- 1/2 tsp garlic powder
- 1/2 cup 2 tbsp blanched almond flour
- 1 tbsp oat fiber
- 1/2 tsp xanthan gum
- 1 tsp baking powder
- 1 tsp active dry yeast
- 2 tbsp hot (~110F) water, also such as dissolving yeast
- Two large eggs (just one for bread, one for Egg wash)
- 1 tbsp coconut (or coconut) Flour, for instance dough

Filling

- 1 1/2 cups keto spinach dip
- 1 oz shredded cheddar or mozzarella
- 2 tbsp grated parmesan

Directions

- Preheat oven to 375F. Get 9" round skillet by completely marring, or even a baking sheet with lining with parchment paper (see previously).
- Apply yeast to warm water and let dissolve, stirring to break up any clumps.

- Sift together dry ingredients (almond milk, oat fiber, xanthan gum, baking powder, and garlic powder, Italian seasoning).

- In a microwave-safe bowl, combine shredded cheeses, cream cheese, and butter. Microwave for 60-90 minutes, or till cheese is melted. Stir to blend.

- Add dry ingredients, 1 egg, and yeast mixture into melted cheese mix and blend well until dough forms a ball. Turn dough on a level surface sprinkled with all the coconut bread and simmer lightly, 15-20 days or till no more "tacky" to your touch.

- Optional: For best results, cover the dough with a moist cloth and let it rise in a warm place for 10-15 minutes.

- Divide dough into two roughly equal segments, then roll into an ~9" circle.

- Distribute the spinach dip onto one circle of bread, stopping just prior to the borders. Top with shredded cheese and parmesan. Twist another circle of bread on top of the filling.

- Make 12 pieces (such as cutting out a pizza) through the layers of bread, being careful to leave them attached at the middle. Select up each "piece" and twist lightly to ensure the "base" layer of bread is at the top.

- Beat the egg and then evenly brush the exposed dough with the egg wash.

- Bake in the preheated oven for approximately 25 minutes, or till golden brown. Optionally, brush with melted butter before serving.
- Best served hot. Store refrigerated for up to 5 times. Reheat in the microwave in the oven in a reduced (~250F) temperature.

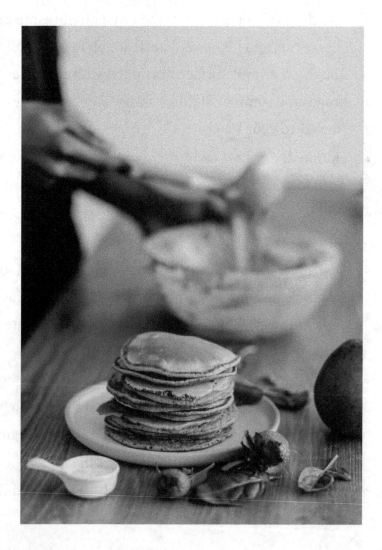

9. Pesto Pull-Apart Keto Bread

This low carb pesto extract bread Is fantastic for your dinner this celebration season, or you'll be able to freeze and it creates a fantastic keto bite for work lunches.

You Don't Have to play tug of war on this One however, there is lots for everybody! It is so badly great it would fool any carbohydrate loving bread blossom to believing it is the real thing! The pesto makes it totally delicious. Served as is stuff with your favorite keto filling. Simple Mediterranean tastes such as tomato and avocado work very nicely with it.

Tips & Substitutions

- Lukewarm water in this recipe may slow down the increasing impact of baking soda. I attempted both heated water and succulent and even though it made no real difference for baguettes, a few individuals have been suffering from air bubbles / hollow interiors after creating a loaf. More information on the best loaf are recorded here.
- To get a paleo, dairy-free choice, try out this almond milk kefir recipe rather than the buttermilk: Use half the almond kefir and half of the water. As an alternative, you

may use the dough to get Ultimate Keto Buns or even Nut-Free Keto Buns (the two recipes have been dairy-free).

- Be certain that you utilize a kitchen scale to measuring all of the dry ingredients. Applying just cups might not be adequate to achieve best outcomes, particularly in baked products. Weights per cups and tsp can fluctuate based upon the product/ manufacturer or whenever you create you have ingredients (such as flax meal out of flaxseeds). Psyllium absorbs a lot of water. When baking using psyllium, you need to be sure to drink enough water during the day to stop constipation!

- It's possible to use some other pesto recipes, such as dairy-free and nut-free choices.

Ingredients

Keto Bread:

- 1 recipe Sourdough Keto Baguettes
- 2/3 cup pesto, you can make your own pesto (170 g/ 6 oz)
- 1/2 cup grated Parmesan or alternative Italian hard cheese (45 g/ 1.6 oz)
- Basil & Arugula Pesto:
- 1/2 cup almonds or pecans (50 g/ 1.8 oz)
- 1 bunch fresh basil (28 g/ 1 oz)

- 2 cups arugula (20 g/ 0.7 oz)
- 4 cloves garlic, chopped
- 2 teaspoon lemon zest
- 1 tablespoon lemon juice (15 ml)
- 1/4 cup extra virgin olive oil
- Sea salt and pepper, to taste

Directions

- Preheat the oven at exactly 170 °C (conventional oven), or 150 °C/ / 300 °F (fan assisted oven).
- To make pesto, put each the ingredients except olive oil into a food processor. Blend till smooth. You are going to want only 2/3 cup of this pesto (or utilize less or more to taste). Any leftover pesto may be saved in the refrigerator and utilized in zucchini noodles along with other keto recipes.
- Ready the bread by following this recipe. Form the dough into rolls (I created 12) however you might easily create 9 larger ones if you would like.
- Spoon about 1 tablespoon of pesto to the middle of every bread roll and then work it in the dough together with your hands on. Roll into chunks.
- Grease an oven proof skillet with just a small coconut butter or oil to prevent sticking.

- Arrange the rolls into a round pattern to approximately cover the bottom of the pan. They'll enlarge on cooking.
- Sprinkle with Parmesan. I don't incorporate the Parmesan from the pesto since I needed on top.
- Bake for 50-60 minutes till golden and cooked throughout. Once completed, remove from the oven and allow the bread cool for 5 minutes.

Tips

To prevent the bread from becoming Moist move from the skillet into a cooling. Tastes best when served hot. Once chilled can be saved in the refrigerator for up to 3 days, or freeze up to 3 weeks.

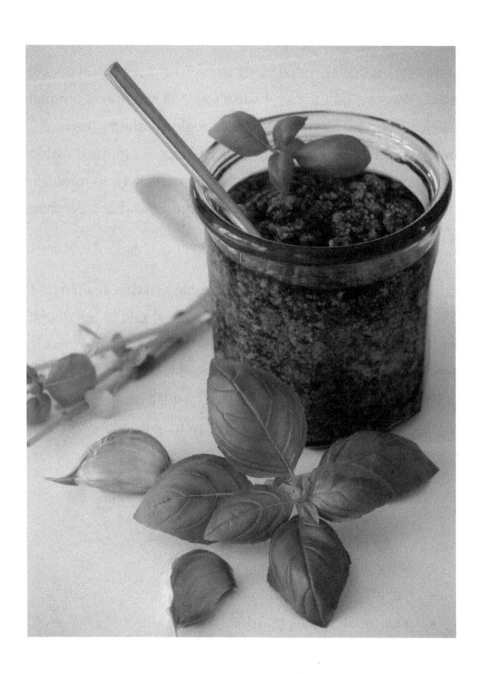

10. Nut Free Keto Rolls

With this particular recipe along with Citrus seed flour you will need floor psyllium husks. I wasn't able to discover a product labeled floor psyllium husk in my regional shops. Instead I purchased the entire psyllium husk and mixed a few fast within my Blendtec blender. I mixed it for approximately 20 minutes. It was not however a wax and it had been somewhat nicer than if it began.

To make this recipe much more enjoyable and Give it a flavor, I included the famed everything but the bagel mix in the dough and in addition to the rolls. Eventually to make them really everything I grated cheese on the top. I'd half cheddar and half of Parmesan cheese. Both were yummy, which means you've got a great deal of alternatives in the event you choose to add yogurt. It's surely optional.

Ingredients

- 120 g of sunflower seed milk
- 5 tbsp of ground psyllium husk
- 2 teaspoon baking powder
- 1/2 teaspoon salt
- 1 plus 1/4th cup boiling water

- 2 teaspoon apple cider vinegar
- 1 tbsp everything but the bagel Seasoning + one tbsp for those shirts
- 3 Egg whites- that I utilized organic ones Out of a carton, therefore I do not need to discover a use for those yokes. In the event you utilize whites out of the carton its own 6 tbsp.

Grated cheese for those shirts is discretionary.

Directions

- Pre-heat oven to 350 plus a baking sheet with parchment
- Mix your sunflower seed bread, ground psyllium husk, baking powder, seasoning and salt in a bowl and whisk until blended
- Add the water and blend for approximately a minute. You might want to change into a spatula or wooden spoon rather than a jolt now.
- Add apple cider vinegar and then blend again.
- Eventually when the mixture has cooled a little put in the egg whites into the bowl. The mixture will probably be well shaped and it could appear the eggs whites will not include - just keep folding and mixing. Kneed the dough together with greased palms until all is integrated. It will not take long.

- With greased hands shape 6 balls. The dough is rather loose and somewhat tacky but you're still able to create chunks.
- Sprinkle your seasoning on the top and push it so it sticks out.
- Cook in the oven for 45 minutes - remove from oven and top with cheese if needed then bake the rest 15 minutes
- Let completely cool before cutting!
- Store in an airtight compartment in your refrigerator.

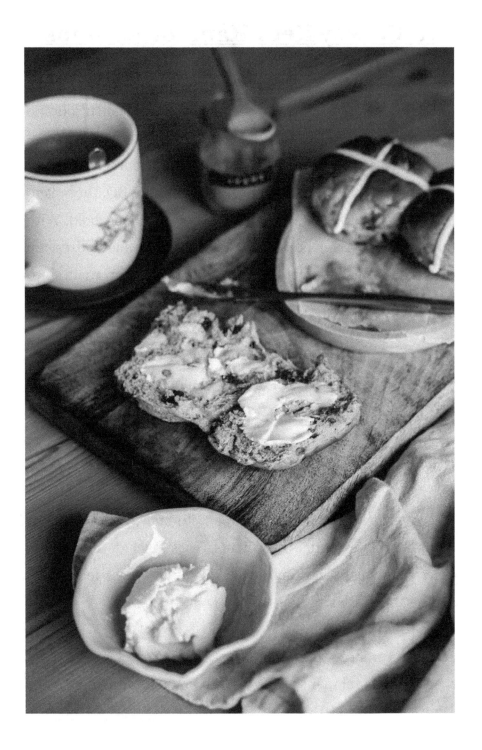

11. Cheesy Keto Hamburger Buns

Tired of serving hamburgers in lettuce wraps? Then look no more. All these keto hamburger buns would be an ideal companion into a tasty, succulent, grass-fed burger. Whether you are enjoying a low-carb meal for a family BBQ, those keto buns will shortly become a staple in your own household. With this keto hamburger bun recipe, then it is possible to dress up your hamburgers any way you'd like: Smother them into sautéed mushrooms, onions, and Swiss cheese. Cover pickles, avocado, red onion, and tomato. Or toast them top with eggs and bacon for a tasty breakfast sandwich. All these keto buns will be the finishing touch on any hamburger -- regardless of how you serve it.

How to Make Keto Hamburger Buns

To create these low fat, gluten-free Keto buns, you're going to require a few essential ingredients. These include mozzarella cheese, cream cheese, almond milk, legumes, grass-fed butter, and sesame seeds.

To begin, preheat your oven at exactly 400° F. Line a baking sheet with parchment paper or coconut oil, and then place aside.

Put in a large bowl, mix your Mozzarella and cream cheese, then microwave for 5-10 minutes, or until the cheese is completely melted.

Insert your eggs into the mixing jar and Combine thoroughly. Ultimately, include the sole tender component (almond milk) into the bowl and then blend again.

With both hands, mould your dough into six chunks in a bun form, then put in your baking sheet. Brush all your low carb buns with butter along with your very last egg. Then sprinkle with sesame seeds. Bake until golden brown, or about 10-12 minutes.

Could this recipe be created dairy-free?

Regrettably, no. As You could Brush every dough ball using olive oil rather than butter, the 2 tsp in this recipe are far overly tricky to substitute a dairy-free alternate.

Could coconut milk be used rather than almond flour?

Sorry, however. Unlike "regular" Baking, in which wheat bread and white bread may be substituted for another in a 1:1 ratio, baking using low-fat recipes is totally different. Grain-free flours like almond, jojoba, flaxseed, and psyllium husk powder have different chemical makeups, and can't be substituted for another.

Can this recipe overeat?

Yes. Should you assess the nutrition details Below, you are going to see these low carb buns are totally free of sugar.

May this recipe be utilized to make Additional keto baked products?

Absolutely. You are able to mould this dough to bagels, bread rolls, as well as keto bread (though you might need to double the ingredients). You might also add a low-carb sweetener into the dough to produce low carb blueberry muffins.

Health Benefits of Keto Hamburger Buns

If you assess that the supplements Information below, you are going to find these ketogenic, low-fat hamburger buns include only 287 calories, which are packed with protein and fat, and contain only 2.4 g of net carbohydrates. Lucky for you, they also include several hidden health advantages.

1: **They Keep You Away from Terrible Foods**

Most store-bought bread goods are Packed with processed flour and unnecessary ingredients. Making these low-fat burger buns from scratch means that you can bypass the additives and fillers.

What does absorbing low-carb bread And bypassing processed goods -- mean to your health? For starters, there's a direct correlation between the use of refined grains as well as the prevalence of type 2 diabetes in the United State.

Second, research indicates a Link between the use of processed foods and an increased risk of celiac disorder. There is a well-established connection between the health of your intestine and also the health of your immune system, also eating processed foods can damage your gut liner. This, then, creates the ideal atmosphere for autoimmunity.

2: **They Are a Fantastic Source of Magnesium**

Magnesium is a Vital mineral That supports almost every significant role within the human body, however the majority of individuals do not get rid of it[*]. This recipe includes two excellent sources of calcium -- sesame seeds and seeds.

Low calcium levels have been connected to type 2 diabetes, metabolic syndrome, elevated inflammation markers, cardiovascular disease, migraine headaches, as well as osteoporosis. Cells low in calcium may even activate systemic inflammation, that is the main cause of almost every contemporary metabolic disorder -- no harm, virus, or bacteria necessary.

Altogether, magnesium includes an Essential part in over 300 cellular responses. However, this active nutrient has to be vaccinated regularly, so be certain that you find these keto burger buns on your meals turning.

3: They Can Help Stabilize Blood Sugar

All these keto hamburger buns are stuffed with nourishment and free of ingredients which may spike your blood glucose. In reality, a few ingredients used in this recipe might help reduce your blood sugar levels.

By Way of Example, CLA (conjugated linoleic Acid) -- that can be found in jojoba oil is a fatty acid that has been proven to enhance insulin sensitivity [*]. Healthful insulin amounts keep blood glucose in check, thus preventing type 2 diabetes and other ailments.

Almonds are just another ingredient Tailor-made for blood glucose management -- and this recipe also includes three cups of these. Almonds are high in healthy fats, calcium and dietary fiber. 1 study found that almond intake improved blood sugar and lipid profiles in several individuals with diabetes

Ingredients

- 2 cups mozzarella cheese (shredded)
- 4 oz. cream cheese
- 4 large eggs
- 3 cups almond milk
- 4 tablespoons. melted grass-fed butter
- Sesame seeds

Directions

- Preheat oven to 400°F.
- Line a baking sheet with parchment paper.
- In a big bowl, mix mozzarella and cream. Heat in the microwave for about 10 minutes, or until both cheeses are melted.
- Add 3 eggs into your cheese mix, and stir to blend. Insert your almond milk, then stir.

- Form dough into 6 bun-shaped balls then put on baking sheet.
- Whisk your very last egg. Brush each dough ball with butter along with your own toaster egg, then sprinkle with sesame seeds.
- Bake until golden, approximately 10-12 minutes.

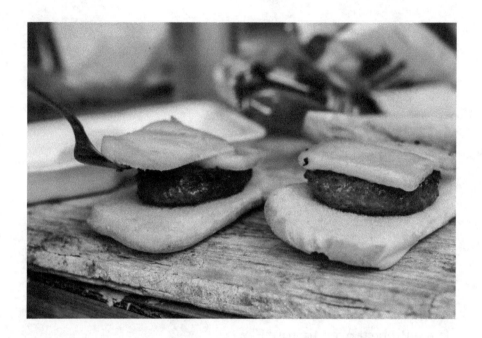

12. Parmesan and Tomato Keto Buns

Fill with your favorite Supply of Keto protein, such as some wonderful broiled chicken with rocket, or even some fantastic older Keto burger. If you enjoy olives, you may even try mixing a few from the batter together with the sun-dried berries. Would totally do the job.

Ingredients
Dry ingredients:

- 3/4 cup almond milk (75 g/ 2.7 oz)
- 2 1/2 tablespoon psyllium husk powder (20 G / 0.7 oz)
- 1/4 cup coconut milk (30 g/ 1.1 oz)
- 1/4 cup packaged cup noodle meal (38 grams / 1.3 ounce)
- 1 teaspoon cream of tartar or apple cider vinegar
- 1/2 teaspoon baking soda
- 2/3 cup grated Parmesan cheese or Additional Italian hard cheese (60 g/ 2.1 oz)
- 1/3 cup sliced sun-dried tomatoes (37 g/ 1.3 ounce)
- 1/4 to 1/2 tsp pink sea salt.

- 2 tablespoons sesame seeds (18 grams / 0.6 ounce) - Or use two tbsp sunflower, flax, poppy seeds, or 1 tablespoon caraway seeds.

Wet ingredients:
- 3 big egg whites
- 1 big egg
- 1 cup boiling water (240 ml/ 8 fl Ounce)

Note: You're able to make 5 regular/large Buns according to recipe up or down to 10 little buns.

Directions

- Preheat the oven at exactly 175 °C. Utilize a kitchen scale to quantify all of the ingredients and put them into a mixing jar (besides the sesame seeds that are employed for topping): vanilla milk, coconut milk, skillet, psyllium husk powder, and cream of tartar and baking soda, and salt, parmesan cheese and sun-dried tomatoes. Mix all of the ingredients together.
- Add the egg whites and whites and procedure well with a mixer before the dough is thick the reason why you should not utilize just whole eggs would be the buns would not grow with a lot of egg yolk in. Do not squander them use them for creating Home-made Mayo, Easy Hollandaise Sauce or Lemon Curd.

- Add boiling water and process until well blended.

- With a spoon, split the keto buns blend into roll and 5 into buns with your palms. Set them onto a skillet tray or onto parchment paper. They'll expand in proportion, so be certain that you leave some distance between them. You may even utilize little sour trays.

- Top all those buns with sesame seeds (or some other seeds) and lightly push them in the dough, which means they do not fall out. Put in the oven and cook for approximately 45 - 50 minutes until golden on top.

- Remove from the oven, then allow the tray cool and set the buns onto a stand to cool to room temperature.

- Enjoy like you want regular bread with butter, cheese or ham!

- Store at a Tupperware for 2-3 weeks or freeze up to 3 weeks.

Allergy-free Strategies & Suggestions

If for any reason you can not get this Recipe to function, below are a few hints which may help.

- If building a loaf rather than buns, inhale for 75 seconds. Don't utilize a silicon loaf pan - utilize a metallic one rather.

- Allergy-friendly choices: flax-free, multipurpose bread (contains a nut-free alternative), nut-free keto buns (contains flax meal), psyllium-free buns (contain flax meal and nuts).

- In the event you do not need to use coconut milk: Though I have not tried it, then I would use double the total amount of almond milk or flax meal rather than coconut milk (1 cup of almond milk / flax meal rather than 1/2 cup coconut bread). Or you can use the Identical amount but Decrease the water from ~ 1/2 cup

- For optimum results, use a kitchen when measuring all of the dry ingredients. Applying just cups might not be adequate to achieve best outcomes, particularly in baked products. Weights per cups and tsp can fluctuate based upon the product/ manufacturer or whenever you create you have ingredients (such as flax meal out of flaxseeds). Psyllium absorbs a lot of water.

- Cream of tartar and baking soda behave as leavening agents. This is the way it works: To receive 2 tsp of fermented coconut powder, then you will need 1/2 a tsp of baking soda plus one tsp of cream of tartar. In the event that you there is no cream of tartar, then rather it is possible to use apple cider vinegar.

- When baking using psyllium, you need to be sure to drink enough water during the day to stop constipation!

- I have had best results using psyllium husks I wax myself. Store-bought readymade psyllium powder might lead to dense buns.

- In case the last outcome is overly moist, don't lessen the water used in this recipe or so the psyllium will clump. Rather, wash the buns from the oven at low up to 100 °C/ / 210 °F for 30-60 minutes. If necessary, cut in half and set into a toaster.

- Don't leave the batter beyond the oven for a long time. Put in the oven once you type the buns.

- For more advice about the best way best to bake the best keto bread, then have a look at the troubleshooting inside this recipe.

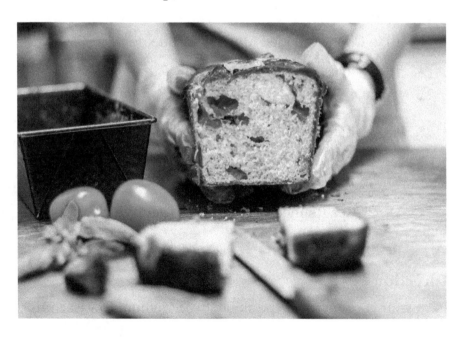

13. Indian Fry Bread

Spicy fried low carbohydrate bread fried into a golden brown, then topped with your favorite taco toppings to get an Indian bake bread taco! This recipe is a very low carb, keto, gluten free. The real key to creating these works would be to NOT overcook them. They only require about 20 minutes of skillet every side. They're somewhat flimsy to utilize, so I advise having a set of long tongs. This way you may get a grasp on the full bake bread to reverse it over in the pan. And they are a little oily, but that is how fry bread will be!

Ingredients

- 1 1/2 Cups Shredded Mozzarella Cheese
- Two Tablespoons Cream Cheese
- 1 Egg
- 1 Teaspoon Baking Powder
- 1 Cup Almond Flour or you can utilize Reduce Wholesome Mama Baking Blend
- 1 1/2 Cups Refined Coconut Oil to get frying

Directions

Heat your coconut oil in the skillet over Medium-low warmth.

Create the Dough:

- At a large skillet, melt Mozzarella cheese and curry.

- Stir then add lemon and egg Powder and stir.

- Add almond milk, 1/4 cup at a time, stirring well after each addition. (You ought to possess a much, homogenous dough. You might need to knead it with your hands somewhat.)

- Turn dough on parchment paper and Split into four chunks.

- Flatten each ball involving parchment Paper and roll into a 6-8 inch ring using a rolling pin.

Fry the Dough:

- After the oil gets warmed, fry dough (one at a time) for approximately 20 minutes, then reverse and simmer 20 minutes on the opposing side. The bread needs to be a light golden brown colour.

- Evacuate from the oil then drain on paper towels.

- Serve with taco toppings for an Indian Fry Bread Taco!

Notes

(These bake breads are best when consumed Immediately after ingestion.)

Nutritional advice is for fry Bread just (not toppings).

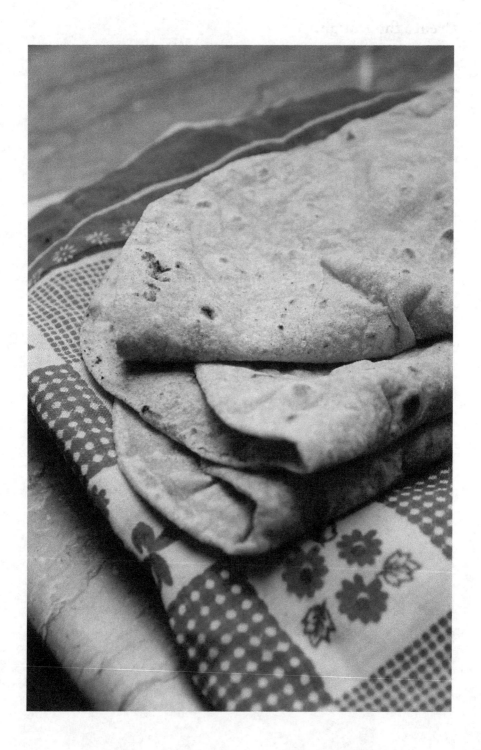

14. Keto Naan Bread

This keto naan with vanilla milk Recipe is produced out of a spin onto my fathead pizza bread recipe. I enjoy using fathead dough to get low carb bread replacements since it's a chewy texture, making it look so much like the greater carbohydrate versions. We knead together the fathead curry recipe. When it includes put it into a ball and then we will divide into six segments -- use a knife to cut as a pie.

We then roll them into chunks and shape Them to the naan contours and inhale.

PRO TIP: Keto naan bread has been intended to get a rustic silhouette, therefore it does not have to be perfectly around, or totally shaped. I believed it was simpler to simply shape with my hands in the utilize a rolling pin, but if you really do need to roll it out, then be certain that you use parchment paper on either side of this naan so it does not adhere to the rolling snare.

When it is done baking and contains Beautiful gold spots around, it is time to find the best area! This keto flatbread is wrapped with an addicting mix of butter, garlic, and parsley. Do not even consider skipping this component!

Keto naan bread really is really a low carb flatbread. Conventional naan is an oven-baked flatbread that's found in several Asian and Indian cuisines, but it is made out of flour and undoubtedly isn't low carb or keto.

How Many Carbs in Keto Naan?

1 Part of keto naan contains only 6 Grams net carbohydrates. Wonderful, right? Conventional naan bread includes over 40 g carbs.

Can You Freeze Low Carb Naan?

It's true, it is possible to freeze low-carb naan. There are two practical strategies to get this done.

Create the dough, form a ball Gradually in plastic, and then freeze it. If you would like to utilize it, then allow it to thaw completely then form into naan bits. Bake as usual.

Pre-bake that the keto naan bread. I Prefer this choice for advantage -- no thawing required! Bake the naan as guided, wrap it, and then store in the freezer. Whenever you're all set to enjoy that, just put in the garlic butter and bake for a couple more minutes.

Ingredients

- 3 cups Mozzarella cheese
- 2 tablespoon Full-fat Greek yogurt
- 2 large Eggs
- 1 1/2 cups Blanched almond milk
- 1 tablespoon Gluten-free baking powder
- 2 tablespoon Butter
- 1/2 tsp Garlic powder
- 1 tablespoon Fresh parsley (chopped)

Directions

- Preheat the oven at exactly 375F. Line additional big baking sheet with parchment paper.
- Combine the shredded mozzarella and Greek yogurt into a huge bowl. Microwave for 2-3 minutes, stirring every 30 minutes, until melted and stirrable to become eloquent. Stir again in the conclusion until well integrated. (you might also use a double boiler on the stove in case you would like.
- In a skillet, stir together the vanilla milk, baking powder, as well as egg whites.
- Working fast while the cheese is still warm, add the pasta mixture into the cheese mix. Knead with your hands through your palms, until a dough form.

- Form the dough into a ball. When it's tacky, cool in the fridge for approximately 15 minutes, only until slightly cool to the touch but not inflexible or icy cold. (It is optional, just if it's too awkward to use)

- Cut the dough ball to 6 segments, like a pie. Take 1 slice, roll into a ball, and then form with your palms into a flatbread contour, roughly 1/4 inch (6 mm) thick.

- Bake the naan from the oven for approximately 8 to 11 minutes, before some gold brown stains shape, however slightly before it appears completely done. If any bubbles shape, pop them using a fork.

- In a small bowl, whisk together the butter, garlic powder and fresh carrot. Brush within the Naan.

- Return the naan into the oven for approximately two minutes, until longer gold brown.

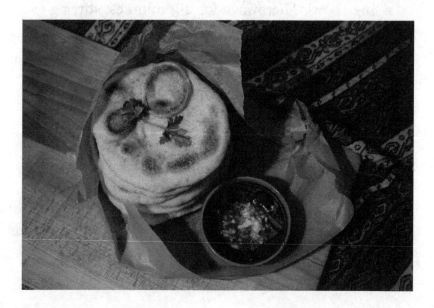

Keto Bread Recipes to Satisfy Sweet Cravings

Though Your cravings for candy treats Should deteriorate following the 30-day markers of beginning a ketogenic diet, it is normal for a few to linger. You might even encounter this, a few months in your trip using a random urge for candy spectacular from the blue. As Opposed to give to a cheat day, try these recipes to satisfy your sweet flavor buds without even undermining weeks of work:

15.Sugar-Free Keto Banana Bread Recipe

This Low-carb banana bread recipe with almond milk & coconut milk is totally moist & abundant. Nobody will know it is keto banana bread! Obviously, paleo, fermented, sugar free, and wholesome.

For the longest time, it appeared as Though developing a low-carb banana bread recipe has been improbable. And that was miserable.

After all you would not have the ability to Include banana at a keto banana bread too many carbohydrates. And without it, then you would miss the point entirely.

But it came! There's a Way to consume perfectly moist and tasty, fermented sugar-free banana bread with no causing anything (except that the carbohydrates). Yay!

Dairy-Free Substitution

You can create this Low-carb banana Bread recipe dairy-free should you want to. The two ghee and coconut oil will be potential dairy-free options into this called-for butter.

Considering that the recipe requires creaming the butter, the final result will probably be somewhat different. However, it will still do the job!

Use Fresh Baking Powder

I know your baking powder Is not bad. However, if it has been at the cupboard since who-knows-when, odds are that it is really time to purchase a few new.

Keto banana bread does not rise very Well, so refreshing baking soda is particularly important to allow it to grow as far as you can.

An Option for Improving Texture

If you do not mind using xanthan gum, then Adding 1/2 tsp to the dry ingredients will produce the feel simpler and stronger. It is not mandatory, however.

Round the Top

Since it doesn't grow much, forming the batter by supplementing the shirt will assist your low carb banana bread recipe appear more conventional.

Consider Covering It Part Way Through

Keep an eye on your bread because it bakes and contemplate covering the best when desired.

How can you know that your sugar-free Banana bread requires this piece of TLC? If the top begins to brown but also the interior remains moist, that is when you pay it. Straightforward tent that the shirt with foil and continue baking your banana bread till it is completed.

Be Patient

If you have been studying a Great Deal of low Carb recipes about here, you are going to see me say that patience ought to be included as part of the majority of recipes. And it is so difficult!

As eager as you can dive into Your fermented sugar-free banana bread, waiting till it is cool is vital if you do not want it to fall apart.

How to store

Are you prepared to get sour? You can Go right ahead and create a double batch if you would like, as this low-carb banana bread recipe keeps well.

It'll Be fine for a Few days on the countertop, and you are able to keep it in the refrigerator for much longer. If you are likely to wash it, then wrap in parchment paper rather than plastic, so it does not accumulate a lot of. Moisture and make soggy.

It is going to also freeze well. Just Slice this up and suspend the pieces. This way it is possible to pull it out since you wish to utilize it!

That is a joyous and fantastic low Carb vacation recipe to talk with your friends because nobody will realize it is keto banana bread, or give as a present to your fellow low-carb, sugar-free enjoying pals.

Ingredients

- 2 cup Blanched almond milk
- 1/4 cup Coconut flour
- 1/2 cup Walnuts (chopped; and much more for instance if desired)
- 2 teaspoon Gluten-free baking powder
- 2 tsp Cinnamon
- 1/4 teaspoon Sea salt (optional)
- 6 tablespoon Butter (softened; may utilize Coconut oil to dairy-free, however taste and texture will differ)
- 1/2 cup Allulose
- 1/2 tsp Xanthan gum
- 4 large Egg
- 1/4 cup Unsweetened almond milk
- 2 tsp Banana infusion

Directions

- Preheat the oven at exactly 350F. Line a 9x5 at (23x13 cm) loaf pan with parchment paper, so the paper pops over two different sides (for simple removal afterwards).
- In a big bowl, combine together the almond milk, coconut milk, baking powder, cinnamon, and sea salt (if using).
- In another bowl, utilize a hand mixer to butter and simmer until fluffy. Beat in the eggs (use the minimal setting to prevent splashing). Stir in the banana extract and vanilla milk.
- Pour the dry ingredients to the wet. Rely on low setting before a dough/batter form.
- Stir in the chopped peppers.
- Put your batter into the lined loaf pan and press evenly to make a smooth surface. When desired, sprinkle the surface with extra chopped peppers and then press them gently to the surface.
- Bake for about 60 minutes, until an inserted toothpick comes out clean.
- Cool completely before evacuating from the pan and then trimming. (The more you allow it to sit before clipping, the greater it will take together. The following day is perfect if at all possible.)

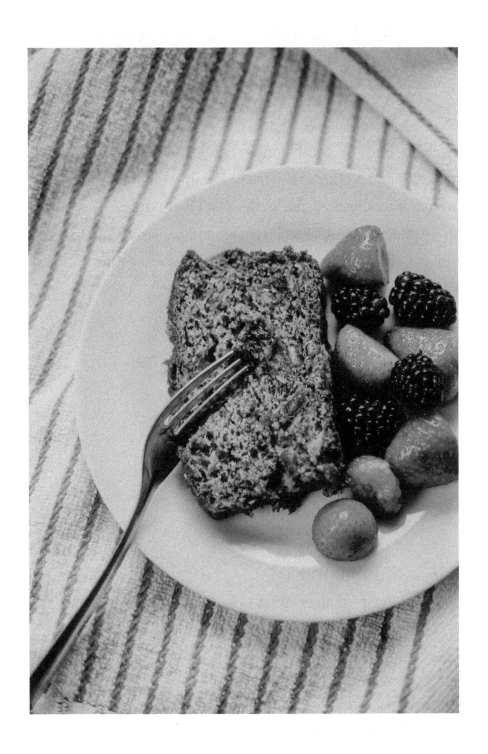

16. Low-Carb Gluten-Free Blueberry Crumb Loaf

A moist and flavorful coffee cake Loaf baked with fresh tomatoes and a cinnamon streusel crumb topping! The feel of the loaf is totally ideal, due to this Oat Fiber I utilize. It provides an extremely cake-like feel without adding carbohydrates, just a lot of fiber! And be mindful, brands do issue together with Oat Fiber.

Ingredients
- 1 3/4 cups super nice almond flour
- 1/4 cup Oat Fiber
- 2/3 cup blueberries
- 3 eggs
- 1/2 cup sour cream
- 1/4 cup thick cream
- 1/2 cup swerve confectioners
- 2 tsp baking powder
- 1 1/2 tsp vanilla extract
- zest of 1 lemon
- Pinch of salt

For the Crumb Topping

- 2/3 cup super-nice almond flour
- 3 tablespoons walnuts, sliced
- 3 tbsp grass fed butter, melted
- 1/4 teaspoon ground cinnamon
- 1/4 cup Brown Swerve
- 1/8 teaspoon ground nutmeg

Directions

- Preheat oven to 325F.
- Add all of the ingredients to the crumb Topping into a bowl except the egg and blend together.
- Add your melted butter then blend Until blended, then put aside.
- Add the flour, baking powder, oat Salt and fiber into a bowl and mix together, then put aside.
- Then add all of the rest Ingredients, except the nourishment into a large mixing bowl and blend using a hand mixer for approximately 30 minutes.
- Add the dry ingredients and Continue blending.
- Fold in the blueberries softly, then Pour into a 9" x 5" nonstick loaf pan that has been sprayed together with nonstick spray (I used coconut oil spray). If your pan is not nonstick, I'd line it with parchment paper. Smooth the top with your spatula and top with the reserved crumb topping.

- Bake for 45-50 minutes, when inserted, comes out clean.

Note:

The Oat Fiber is also Crucial in This recipe! I use it so many recipes, due to the wonderful texture it provides everything I'm baking! It's upside down, the ideal ingredient I have baked together and is actually worth purchasing. I utilize Life source Foods Oat Fiber 500 since they grind it into a very good powder also has a mild taste. I purchase it at the 16 ounce bag. The bag lasts some time, since you don't have to use much on your own recipes.

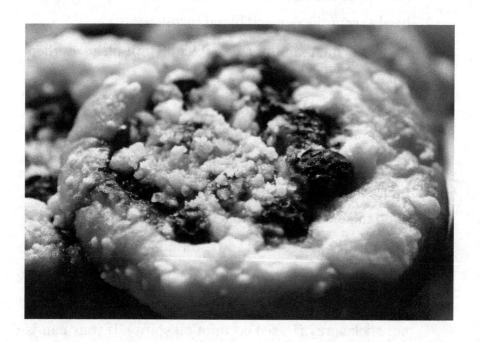

17. Keto Lemon "Poppy Seed" Bread Loaf

Everybody likes Starbucks and they have Got some very yummy things. We thought we would take one of the tastiest delights and create a Keto edition of this Starbucks Lemon Poppy seed Bread.

It is Gluten Free, Low Carb and only and very yummy. This recipe is very sweet, zesty and incredibly filling. This recipe makes 12 functions. 1 function is 1 piece once the loaf is sliced into 12 pieces. Maintain the Keto Starbucks Lemon Poppy Seed Loaf coated in the refrigerator for up to 1 week or two slit and freeze up to 3 weeks.

Ingredients

- 9.5 oz (3 cups) of Almond Flour
- 1/2 teaspoon of Baking Powder
- 1/2 cup of Sukrin:1 Sweetener
- 2 tbsp of Poppy Seeds
- Two Lemons, zest only
- 3 tbsp of Lemon Juice
- 3 tbsp of Butter, melted
- 6 Eggs

Glaze:

- 1/2 cup of Natvia Icing Mix
- 1 tbsp of Lemon Juice
- 1-2 tbsp of Water

Directions

- Preheat oven to 175C/350F.
- In a big mixing bowl then add your almond milk, and poppy seeds, and baking powder. Mix thoroughly.
- Add the lemon juice, lemon zest and butter then blend well.
- Add the eggs and blend until all united
- Pour the mix in your lined 9×5 loaf.
- Bake in your oven for nearly an hour.
- Permit it to cool for 20 minutes.

Glaze:

- Insert the icing mixture and lemon juice into a small mixing bowl.
- Gradually add the water until the mix has a pouring consistency.
- Sprinkle over the cooled loaf, cut it into 12 pieces and enjoy!

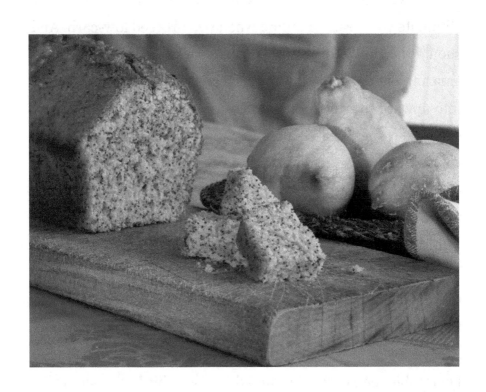

18. Low-Carb Lemon Blueberry Bread

Pairing lemon is Common from the dessert planet. This recipe to get a keto peppermint and lemon loaf (pictured above) may eliminate your fears of falling when you proceed low-carb. And should the combo of sour lemon and sweet polyphenols is not amazing enough, this low carb recipe also sneaks in zucchini into upward the nutritious macros. You will even know how to generate a sugar-free lemon zest to ice your own loaf so that your children are going to enjoy it as far as possible. As you won't actually taste the inclusion of zucchini, you might choose to provide this recipe a try too.

This healthier lemon blueberry zucchini Bread recipe isn't hard to create with 15 seconds prep. A tasty low carb zucchini bread that is gluten-free, sugar free, and paleo!

Lemon blueberry zucchini bread is also a bit Light, summery cake-like bread which utilizes seasonal tastes, comes together only, and is ideal for breakfast, a snack, as well as dessert. This very low carb zucchini bread recipe is more fermented sugar free, and amazingly easy to create. Keto zucchini bread can also be among my absolute preferred ways to use zucchini at a recipe... plus also a fantastic way to finish off Zucchini Week!

This lemon blueberry zucchini bread Recipe really makes my beloved low carb zucchini bread however. And like I said, it is totally a cure. Blueberry zucchini bread with lemon zest is great for dinner, however, it's also healthy enough to lunch! Or like it with some tea or coffee in the day, also.

The zucchini retains it light on the two Calories and carbohydrates, and that means you're able to delight in this very low carb zucchini bread recipe with no guilt in any way. Plus, it tastes so decadent which you can practically call it lemon zucchini cake. Especially when you have children who enjoy cake and wish to sneak a few additional veggies into their own diets.

Ingredients

- 1/2 cup Butter (softened)
- 3/4 cup Erythritol (or some other granulated Length of option)
- 3 large Egg
- 1 tablespoon Lemon juice
- 1 tablespoon Lemon zest (optional)
- 1 teaspoon Vanilla extract
- 2 cup Blanched almond milk
- 2 teaspoon Gluten-free baking powder
- 1/4 teaspoon Sea salt

- 1 1/2 cup Zucchini
- 1 cup Blueberries

Lemon Glaze
- 1/4 cup Erythritol (roasted in a Food chip; or utilize any additional liquid or powdered detergent of choice)
- 4 teaspoon Lemon juice

Directions
- Preheat the oven at exactly 325F. Line a 9x5 at (23x13 cm) loaf pan with parchment paper. (it is possible to use transparency, however dirt nicely.)
- In a big bowl beat the butter and erythritol, until fluffy.
- Beat in the eggs, lemon juice, lemon zest (if using), and vanilla extract.)
- Beat in the almond milk, baking powder, and sea salt.
- Wrap the grated zucchini into cheesecloth or a couple layers of paper towels. Squeeze above the sink to discharge just as much moisture as possible. Squeeze the grated zucchini to the jar, and blend well.
- Fold the blueberries to the batter.
- Transfer the batter into the prepared pan. Smooth the surface with your spoon, then rounding the shirt slightly. Bake for 60-70 minutes, until an inserted toothpick comes out clean. Cool completely in the pan.

- To Create the glaze, conduct the batter by means of a blender to allow it to be powdered. (Or, you can use a powdered sweetener right, such as Erythritol Confectioner's or Sukrin Melis.) Stir together the lemon juice powdered sweetener. Drizzle the glaze over bread.

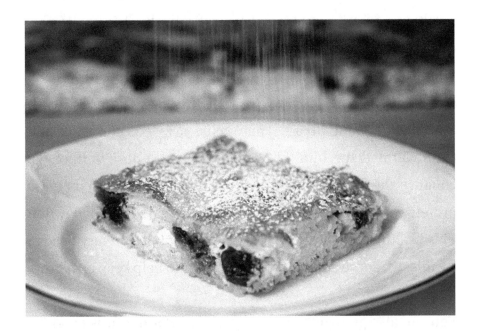

19. Keto Coconut zucchini Bread Together with Pecan

There are so many Low-carb bread Choices for you to pick to a keto diet. Every sort of bread has its own particular taste. You might have tried or heard zucchini bread or even coconut bread but have you tried making them collectively? We create this candy bread for a snack which will go nicely with coffee and tea. You're able to allow it to be a low-carb side for supper by taking away the sweetener. Now we're showing you that our low carb Zucchini Coconut Bread. This recipe uses coconut milk and freshly grated zucchini that delivers an extra dose of fiber. To enhance the feel, add greater consistency and also to increase protein consumption we use 1 scoop of low carb protein powder. This healthy bread is going to keep you complete. Every once in a while, we adore adding protein powder to help keep us plump.

You can also go together with hydration Powder, it is good for skin, hair, nail and nourishment also. Another fantastic news is that hydration is more heat stable, and also kind of tasteless. We are going to be creating more recipes together with hydration later on.

Ingredients

- 3/4 cup coconut milk

- 1/2 cup zucchini (drained and grated)
- 1/4 cup Pecan (sliced)
- 3/4 tablespoon baking powder
- 1 teaspoon vanilla extract
- 1 spoonful unflavored protein powder (approximately 28 - 30g)
- 6 large eggs
- 1/2 cup butter grated
- 1/2 cup Thus Nourished Erythritol (or even Less, up to a liking)
- 1/2 tsp salt

Directions

- Preheat your oven to 350°F.
- Rinse the zucchini nicely with water and then apply a hand grater to fix it. Salt the grated zucchini in a bowl. Proceed to a colander to drain some other fluids that are unnecessary. You need to get about 1/2 cup of drained and shredded zucchini.
- Start creating the dry mix in a bowl. Fold the coconut bread, baking powder and protein powder using the sweetener. Mix until combined entirely.
- Beat the eggs into a mixer with vanilla extract and melted butter. Move the grated zucchini in and carefully insert the dry mix also. Whisk together until integrated. Reduce the chopped pecan.

- Coat a skillet with peanut butter. Evenly disperse the bread batter to the pan. Put in the oven for about 40-45 minutes until the bread is cooked and refrigerated. When the surface turns gold, take away from the oven and let sit 10 minutes before removing from the pan.
- Slice and revel in!

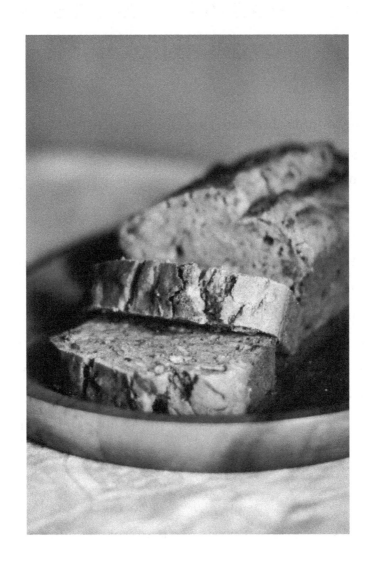

20. Low-Carb Dual Chocolate Zucchini Bread

A yummy double chocolate zucchini Bread that is low carb and gluten free. And it is also super moist as a result of the inclusion of zucchini.

The Traditional way it is made contains a lot of standard sugar. Because of this, there is 20 g of carbohydrates in a tiny slice.

More than half of these grams of carbohydrates come from sugars. Simple sugars, so I am convinced I do not have to remind one, evoke a release of this hormone, insulin. The more frequently insulin is released on your blood to maintain blood glucose in check, the more resistant the cells would be into the endocrine system.

Thus, more than with much more and much simpler sugars absorbed your pancreas has to work to keep up with demand.

Ingredients
- 1/2 cup coconut milk

- 1/2 cup unsweetened cocoa powder
- 1/2 cup Lakanto Golden Monk Fruit Granular Sweetener or routine white
- 1/2 teaspoon ground cinnamon
- 1 tsp baking soda
- 1 tsp baking powder
- 1/4 tsp salt
- 1/4 cup coconut oil fractionated
- 4 large eggs
- 1 tsp vanilla
- 2 cups zucchini stained
- 1/2 cup sugar free chocolate chips

Directions

- In large mixing bowl, combine the coconut milk, cocoa, sweetener, cinnamon and baking soda, baking powder, and salt.
- Blend at the eggs, coconut oil, and vanilla until well blended.
- Fold from the zucchini and chocolate chips.
- Pour mix into a greased or parchment paper lined 9×5-inch loaf.
- Bake in 350°F for about 45-55 minutes or till toothpick inserted near center comes out clean.

- Evacuate from the oven and cool on rack for 15 minutes before removing from pan. Cool thoroughly before slicing.

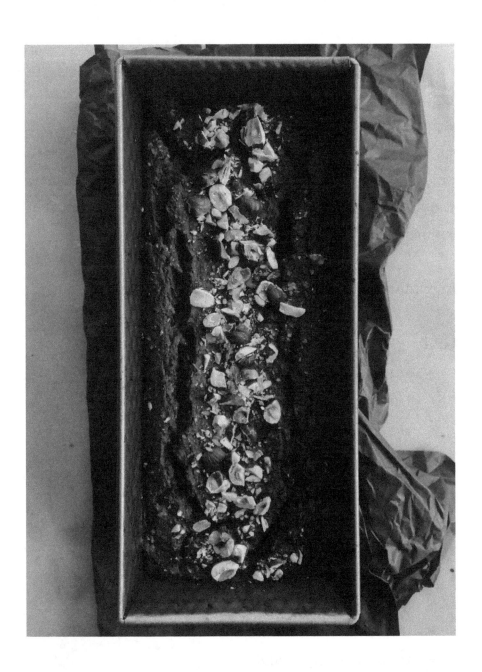

21. Keto Gingerbread Cake

You do not have to await the autumn and winter months to appreciate this keto loaf. And because this Starbucks copycat recipe is 100% sugar free, according to the recipe founders, you may enjoy it without the massive spike in insulin you'd have with all the store-bought edition. The following keto recipe may also be savored yearlong, particularly if you're a lover of pumpkin (and want more than 1 period of this).

Ingredients

Loaf

- 1/2 cup Unsalted Butter softened
- 1/2 cup natvia
- 1/2 tsp vanilla extract
- 4 oz Cream Cheese softened
- 1 large Egg
- 1 1/2 cups almond milk
- 1 1/2 tsp Baking Powder
- 2 tsp Ginger floor
- 1 tsp cinnamon floor
- 1/2 tsp ground
- 1/2 tsp nutmeg ground
- 1 pinch Salt

Frosting

- 4 ounce Cream Cheese softened
- 1 tsp vanilla extract
- 1.5 oz natvia icing mix
- 2 tbsp walnuts chopped

Direction

Loaf

- Preheat your oven to 165C/330F.
- Add the butter Natvia to a stand mixer and beat on medium speed with the whisk attachment.
- Add the cherry, vanilla and cream cheese and then blend.
- In a mixing bowl, then add the rest of the loaf ingredients and blend together.
- Gently fold the dry ingredients to the rack mixer.
- Pour the batter into a 9x5in loaf tin, lined with parchment.
- Bake in your oven for nearly an hour, until a skewer comes out clean when inserted at the middle.
- Permit the loaf to sit at the tin for 15 minutes before removing to a wire cake rack to cool fully

Frosting

- On your rack mixer, blend the cream cheese, vanilla and Natvia Icing Mix. Mix on medium speed till smooth.

- Spread on the cooled loaf and top with the chopped peppers. Cut to 10 pieces and love.

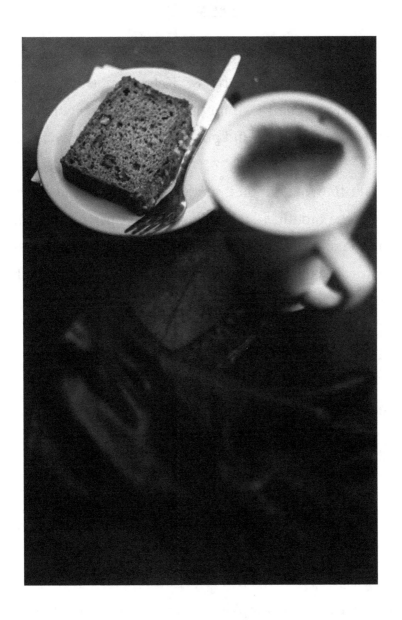

22. Pumpkin and Orange Cheese Bread

This is the best low-carb & Keto recipe for collapse. Straightforward cherry & pumpkin spice roasted curry topped with creamy strawberry and pumpkin cheesecake layers.

The grain-free foundation is tender and moist, while the carrot melts on the mouth. 1 loaf makes 10 to 12 parts based on the magnitude of every cut. Rather than a normal loaf it's possible to create cakes instead. They're better for part management and freeze well.

Ingredients

Cheesecake topping:

- 2 1/2 cups cream cheese (600 grams / 1.3 Pounds)
- 1 large egg
- 1/3 cup roasted Erythritol or Swerve (53 g/ 1.9 oz)
- 1 teaspoon organic orange extract or two tsp Nice orange zest
- 2 tablespoons fresh orange juice (30 ml)
- 1/2 teaspoon pumpkin pie spice mixture or cinnamon

- 1/2 cup unsweetened pumpkin puree (100 grams / 3.5 oz)

Bread:
- 2 cups almond milk (200 g/ 7.1 oz)
- 2 teaspoon pumpkin pie spice mixture (you can Create your own)
- 1 teaspoon cream of tartar or apple cider vinegar
- 1/2 teaspoon baking soda
- 1 tablespoon orange zest
- 1/4 cup of virgin coconut oil
- 4 large eggs
- 1/2 cup of Swerve
- 3/4 cup unsweetened pumpkin puree (150 grams / 5.3 oz)

Directions
- Ready the cheesecake topping. In a bowl, mix the cream cheese, sweeteners, egg, orange extract and orange juice. Optionally, add a couple drops of stevia. Put aside.
- Preheat the oven at exactly 175 °C. In a bowl, mix the dry ingredients: vanilla milk, pumpkin spice blend, cream of tartar and baking soda.
- In another bowl, whisk the eggs, melted butter and simmer. Optionally, add a couple drops of stevia.

- Transfer the egg mix into the bowl with the dry ingredients and blend well. Spoon at the pumpkin puree and blend in.

- Add orange zest (finely grated or approximately just like I'd mine). Optionally, you may add 2 to 4 tablespoons of orange juice. This is going to end in a cake which is moist.

- Spoon your bread batter in a loaf pan (I used 23 x 13 cm/ 9 x 5 inches) and distribute evenly.

- Insert a layer utilizing half the cheese mixture in addition to the chili batter and spread evenly.

- Mix the remaining mixture using all the pumpkin puree and pumpkin pie spice.

- Gently spoon the pumpkin cheese mix on the top and spread evenly. Move to the oven and bake for 50 to 60 minutes. Keep a watch out for the bread, even as it might get burnt in addition to (To stop the cheesecake from cracking, then put a little ramekin full of water to the oven beside the loaf pan)

- Once completed, open the door of the oven and then allow the bread gradually cool down. If it reaches room temperature (1-2 hours), carefully remove from the skillet and then slit.

- Best chilled fully overnight in the refrigerator. It'll allow it to be company and easier to cutback.

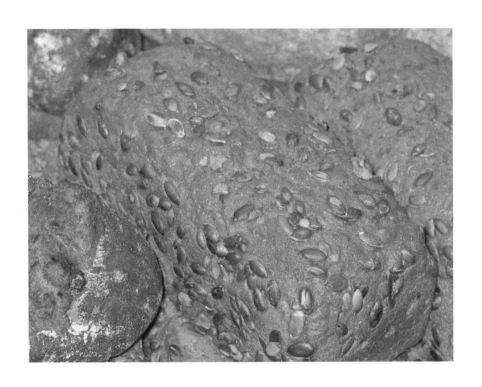

CONCLUSIONS

Carbohydrates have been the Outcasts of this food world - delivered to the courageous step for endangering our waistlines. But they are crucial element of a balanced, healthful diet, critical for any variety of physiological processes to assist us daily.

So regardless of the low carb diet tendency Taking the findings published today verifying that low-fat diets aren't any more powerful than conventional low-carb diets, aren't any surprise. Carbs have been public enemy #1, particularly for those attempting to eliminate weight, but in precisely the exact same time, there is also a great deal of confusion about what they're.

No, milk products, such as butter, are believed fats. But carbohydrates are a far bigger food collection which goes beyond white bread as well as bread.

Today's fad, the keto diet concentrates on high fat, moderate protein and low carbohydrate targeted primarily in the fitness center and weight loss marketplace. It is predicting the keto diet since ketones will be the origin of energy the body uses if it is burning off fat.

In the Brief term, low carbohydrate Diets can be useful for weight reduction. On the other hand, the health consequences of keeping ketosis for lengthy intervals are unknown, particularly on the intestine microbiomes and ought to be supervised by a medical professional such as a dietitian. That said, I have seen a surge of "keto-friendly" goods from the mainstream marketplace over the previous two years such as the baking industry.

Most of Us know that sugar Is Vital For the sweet flavor. But sugar extends past sweetness and can be a significant component for purpose such as color, feel, and nourishment. While I state sugar, I am talking about table sugar (sucrose.) That makes it trickier to make a low-carb bread or baked great. I have seen a few baking disasters since the sugar from the recipe was meddled with. A couple baking organizations are especially focusing on the keto marketplace. Even substituting maple syrup or honey to table sugar generates new interactions which won't behave just like glucose, resulting in rather different results, like utilizing low sugar additives.

Making a shift isn't a simple job. In case you've tried it, you might have come across a few of the most frequent challenges, such as cravings, sluggishness, and brain fog. Additionally, it may be a psychological challenge; resulting in doubts and needs you didn't know where significant for you. However, you don't need to worry anymore! By introducing Keto bread in your diet plan, you can't just encourage your wellbeing and well-being, however, you might also ease in the lifestyle in a means that's less daunting and more prohibitive compared to other options until you.

The more you understand about the Keto diet Generally, the more you're able to know why Keto bread is still an organic food to Incorporate on your eating program. It Might Sound counter-intuitive to add bread into a low-carb eating strategy; nonetheless, Keto bread is very exceptional due to the Ingredients used in creating it. Some areas sell Keto bread baked for You, however, there are lots of unique recipes you may try out to include it in to Your own Keto plans. You Might Have heard people claiming it's "filthy Keto" into Include substitutions on your daily meal plan, for example bread, but as you Read the info presented within this audiobook you may learn not Just the reason it's helpful to incorporate it on your Keto diet plan, but also why it's necessary!